PAIN IS NOT A LIFE SENTENCE

A GUIDE TO UNDERSTANDING AND ELIMINATING CHRONIC MUSCLE, JOINT, AND NERVE PAIN

BRANDON RAMAKKO
DC, MS, DIANM, RMSK, DipIBLM

CONTENTS

INTRODUCTION

"All your problems are from a vitamin D deficiency."

"Turmeric will solve all your problems."

"Just follow this diet."

"Just do this one trick…"

While vitamin D deficiency is common, curcumin (the active ingredient in turmeric) is a potent anti-inflammatory among its other benefits, and some diets may help most people, there is no one trick to fix everyone because everyone's problems are unique and people are allowed to have multiple overlapping problems. The surgeon thinks your problem needs surgery, the nutritionist thinks it is your diet, the chiropractor thinks it is coming from the neck, the physiotherapist thinks you need to stretch more or do more squats, etc. You follow blindly because you don't know any better.

I was like you once. I'm not stupid, but I knew nothing about healthcare. I had years of chronic problems with no solutions. Chronic joint pain, knee locking, throwing my neck out every month or so, and no long-term solutions given to me. If you don't have your health, you don't have anything, so I quit my college teaching job and went to learn healthcare myself. I want to share as much as I can with you so you can help yourself and your loved ones self-manage your conditions or at least be informed when discussing your problems with the healthcare community.

This book could easily be a few thousand pages long to cover all conditions and their solutions, but for practical purposes, this book is focused on the most common neuro-musculoskeletal chronic pain conditions: particularly conditions having a joint, tendon, ligament, or muscular component to them. I do not delve into rare genetic conditions, nutritional deficiencies, or autoimmune conditions, although they should be considered in stubborn chronic cases.

This book is divided into three main parts. The first is useful for everyone to read and is an introduction to what pain is and how pain works along with explanations of common factors in most musculoskeletal chronic pain conditions. The second section is still readable, but may act as more of a resource. It contains lists: healthcare professionals, treatments, common drugs, etc. The third section breaks the body into distinct regions; only a part of the third section might be relevant to the reader depending on the region of their chronic pain.

Even if this book doesn't solve your problems, I have no doubt it will allow you to understand more about your body and may allow you to help the ones you love minimize their pain.

PART 1:
QUESTION AND ANSWER

WHAT/WHY/HOW OF PAIN

Why Pain?

What if we didn't have pain? Without pain, an individual won't realize they've hurt themselves. In the case of sensory loss of the foot, there is a condition called "Charcot foot." They may stub their foot and not realize it. They don't realize that they are injured and they don't make any effort to protect the injury. When it eventually gets X-rayed, the bones are not the right shape and the joints of the foot are not where they should be. So much is wrong at the same time, the radiologist doesn't even know where to begin to describe it: the X-ray looks like a disorganized mess, like an amateur was trying to draw the bones of the foot from memory. These injuries are often amputated.

Think about a hot pan. A hot pan might look the same as a room temperature one. Only pain allows you to tell if something is too hot to handle. We evolved pain for survival. It is ultimately a protection and warning system. If you were designing a protection system, wouldn't you want it to alert you, not only when damage is done, but when damage might occur? Ideally so that you can prevent it? So, our pain system warns us if something might get damaged, informs us if something is damaged, and helps us to protect a damaged region while it heals.

What is Pain?

Pain is something you feel. It is an emotion. It is different in that it has a location component to it but it is an emotion nonetheless.

Where does pain come from?

The pain emotion comes from the same part of the brain that all other emotions come from. However, that isn't the only part of the brain involved in pain. The decision whether to create the pain emotion or not, or how intense it should be, can be a bit complex, but also involves the parts of the brain responsible for memory. This makes sense if you think about it. The pain-related parts of the brain need to remember what is damaged so it can protect that region of the body. It needs to recognize situations that might be dangerous so it knows to listen extra carefully to your senses for danger.

The parts of the brain involved in pain are sometimes referred to as the "pain neuromatrix," but I prefer the term, "pain protection system," as it is more descriptive.

How does pain work?

It first starts with pain sensors. But what is a pain sensor? What does sensing pain mean on a microscopic level? Pain is an emotion, right? There are multiple types of sensors that can ultimately report to the pain processing parts of the brain: high threshold stretch sensors, high threshold temperature sensors, chemical sensors, and sometimes it even includes movement sensors. After you stretch or squish tissue to the point it might get damaged, the high threshold pressure sensors might fire. When you might get burned or freeze, you set off strong signals from temperature sensors. Chemical sensors might register changes in chemistry due to an injury or exertion at the cellular level. And finally, **movement sensors might result in pain to keep you from moving a joint that the body is trying to protect.**

So, the signal then goes straight to the brain for processing, right? Not quite. Some processing happens in the spinal cord. There are neurons (brain cells) in your spinal cord that relay the information up to the brain. Many are surprised to learn that there are many neurons in the spinal cord including the neurons that ultimately end up activating your muscles. The reflexes happen at the level of the spinal cord. When the doctor uses the tiny hammer on your knee tendon that makes the knee do a tiny kick, that happens from the neurons in the spinal cord. The initial, lightning quick, withdrawal from pain happens from these neurons. If it is important to get away, we are designed to pull the limb away before the brain even realizes what is going on. The neurons that relay information up to the brain can alter whether they report to the brain at all and how much they report to the brain. A certain amount of sensor stimulation is required before a signal is sent upwards but that threshold can be changed. Often the threshold for these neurons decreases after an injury as if the body is listening more carefully to the sensors. Once you are healed and safe, the brain can tell these neurons to put the sensitivity back to normal again.

Now the brain gets the signal. What does it do with it? It doesn't just create pain directly proportional to the incoming signal but it modifies the intensity. But what factors does it take to determine how much pain to create? Wouldn't it be useful to know whether a limb is already damaged and/or whether it needs to be extra vigilant? The pain protection system involves the parts of the brain responsible for memory so it uses your memories to try to predict situations where pain may be useful to protect you based on your past experiences. If you have been concerned about your right arm, then your brain is going to amplify any signals involving your right arm. If you have hurt your back before while bending forward, then it might spasm the muscles and send sharp pains to stop you from moving.

You are designed for survival. Often this system goes overboard resulting in overprotection. Better to be alive and in pain rather than dead. The brain can go the other way entirely and turn off pain so that you can run out of the burning building, lift the car off the child, score the winning goal on a sprained ankle, etc.

To summarize, the process of pain starts with sensors which measure temperature, tissue stress, and chemicals. If the signal reaches a threshold, the signal is relayed to the brain by the neurons in the spinal cord. The brain takes into account how much signal is arriving from the spinal cord, your past history/injuries, and your current situation, to determine how much pain you should experience. Pain $\neq$ Damage.

CHRONIC PAIN DISORDERS

Central Sensitization

There are various situations where pain can become chronic or excessive. It is good to keep in mind that Pain ≠ Damage just like cookies ≠ happiness. They can be related but you can have happiness without cookies and the amount of happiness doesn't necessarily correlate to the amount of cookies: plenty of depressed individuals have a box of cookies in their cupboards. When the pain is excessive due to increased **sensitivity** of the **central** nervous system (neurons in spinal cord and the brain) they call it **central sensitization**. In the previous section, I mentioned that the neurons in the spinal cord can develop an increased sensitivity which the brain can reset back to normal levels once the dangerous period is over. But what happens if the danger never ends? The pain system's sensitivity can be ramped up directly by tissue damage or **by the perceived danger** of possible damage.[1] Because of the fear of damage, the pain sensitivity stays high in chronic pain sufferers. Therefore, what would normally be non-painful in a normal individual is painful for them. Moving can become painful, muscles may spasm or remain rigid, touching the surface of the skin can be tender, pain intensity can be severe, and the

---

[1] Quartana PJ, Campbell CM, Edwards RR. Pain catastrophizing: a critical review. *Expert Rev Neurother.* 2009;9(5):745-758. doi:10.1586/ern.09.34

pain can spread out over a larger region. These individuals often fear movement and activities (fear avoidance) and may imagine the worst (catastrophizing). Poor muscle usage results in muscle wasting (atrophy) and tendon degeneration/weakening (tendinosis). Over time the brain forgets how to coordinate more complicated movements increasing the likelihood of them re-injuring themselves. They often develop achy muscles from all the muscle guarding and spasms.

Let's say you visit your doctor after an initial bout of back pain. The doctor tells you not to bend forward or move too fast or you might hurt your back again. He shows you the X-ray/MRI and says the discs are degenerated. "Your back is all worn out." If this is what you hear, your brain may be continuously worried about protecting your back. Some chronic pain sufferers are overly concerned by X-ray or MRI findings and are convinced that their joints are damaged and that further use of their joints will make them worse. But... there are people with degenerative rotator cuff tears, disc bulges, degenerative joint disease (osteoarthritis), vertebral compression fractures (see nearby image), etc. that have ZERO pain. Pain $\neq$ Damage! Not that these issues can't contribute to pain in some people, but seeing them on MRI or X-ray doesn't guarantee pain or, at the very least, doesn't guarantee a lifetime of pain. Also, many chronic pain sufferers have ZERO evidence of tissue injury/damage/degeneration (not that there wasn't an initial injury sometime in the past initiating the chronic pain cycle). The original injury may be healed, but the state of 'high alert' may remain. The brain is not decreasing the sensitivity of the neurons in the spinal cord like it should post-injury, and it may even amplify the pain in a state of fear and protection.

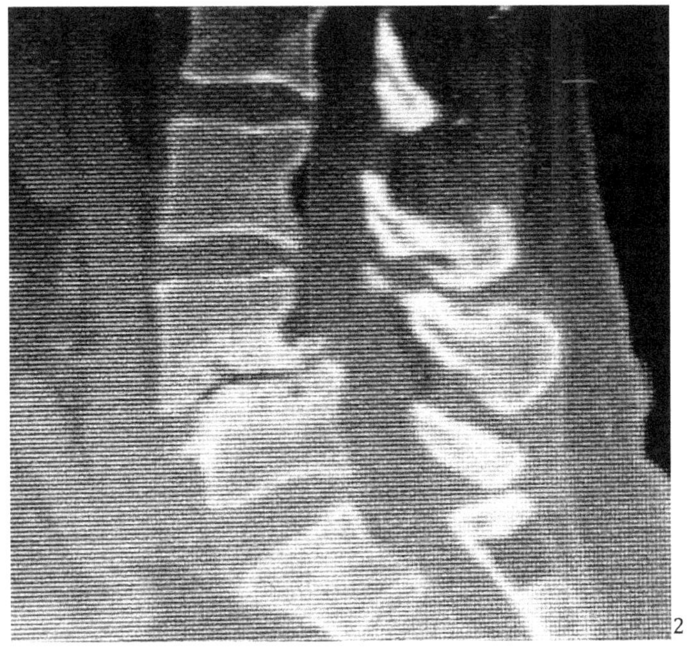

Side note: There is a rarer complication/version of chronic pain syndrome called complex regional pain syndrome (CRPS) where the nervous system messes up things even more, causing the whole injured limb to swell up, change color, change temperature, and change skin/nail texture along with sharply increased pain sensitivity. Most commonly occurs following a fracture or surgery.

---

[2] Used with permission. He did originally have some pain but his healthcare team told him his pain seemed more muscular and to try some exercises for a bit before surgery. This person had no back pain when I was last talking with him despite significant damage seen on the image. He has not had surgery and his favorite activity is golfing and he can swing a club just fine.

How to Help?

Re-frame: pain does not mean damage. Every time there is pain, it does not mean you are doing further damage to your body. Think of the tissues as deconditioned instead of damaged. Deconditioned implies they can be reconditioned again. They can get better and stronger.

Re-map and Re-learn: Through disuse due to fear of pain/damage, the tissues become deconditioned and the brain's ability to properly coordinate the muscles is impaired (use-it-or-lose-it). The brain has a map of the body and it can become smudged and blurry. It doesn't know where the joints are, how fast they are moving, etc. The brain needs to relearn/remap the body. The brain needs to be re-taught how to use the muscles and joints with proper coordination again. Once this is achieved, the brain will have more confidence in using the joints, and there will be reduced risk of future injury/pain.

Physiotherapists, acupuncturists, chiropractors, and massage therapists can all help with the muscle aches and tightness. Physiotherapists, chiropractors, and trainers can help with reconditioning muscles and relearning the body. Psychologists, counselors, hypnotherapists, etc. can help with the central sensitization (brain). Medical doctors can help minimize pain from the sensors through drugs, injections, surgeries, aspirations, nerve ablations, etc., but should be used with caution as the "damage" they see on X-ray or MRI may have nothing to do with your pain, and the drugs may have their own side effects. For more specific strategies, see the fibromyalgia section and/or the region-specific section of the book.

WHAT ARE MUSCLE KNOTS AND HOW DO YOU GET RID OF THEM?

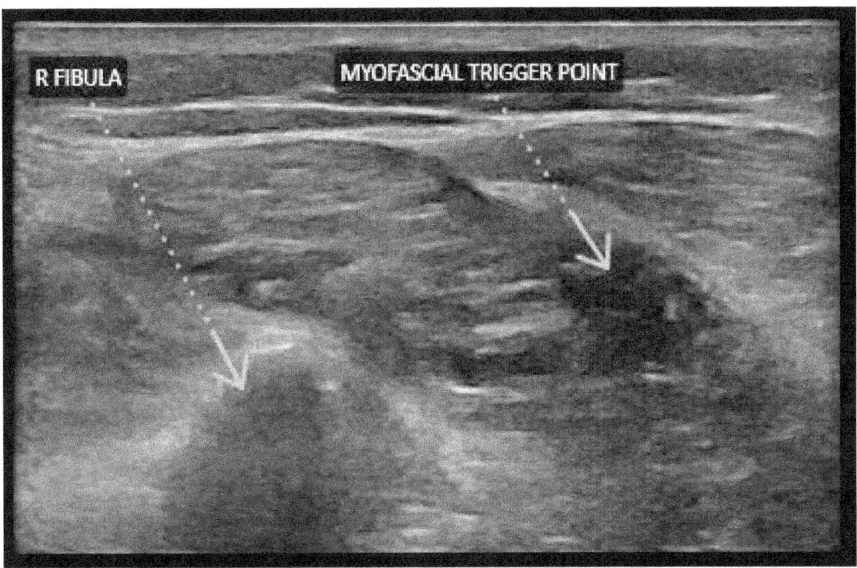

What are they?

Painful muscle knots are also known in medical literature as myofascial trigger points (MFTPs). In my clinical experience everyone has some tender spots in their muscles and individuals may have some tender nodules/knots. It is extremely common to find nastier, more painful knots in those with pain or those who have been injured. The larger and/or more painful nodules often create vague pressure or pain that feels like it spreads out. The pain can be sharper or very dull. The sensation can mimic nerve-type pain and have a slight tingling or burning sensation to it. The pain can be recreated by pushing on the nodule, stretching the muscle, or using the muscle. The nasty muscle knots are partly responsible for all types of chronic pain conditions such as tension-type headaches, hip pain, and shoulder pain.

What causes them?

These muscle knots can form related to stress, an acute injury (an accident), or overuse. They can last for years, so if their creation is related to an injury, they can persist after the injury has healed. Overuse can refer to 'overdoing it,' but in the context of muscle knots, it is more that the muscles may not be sharing the work properly. Using crutches, limping, or developing odd movement patterns can create them. The exact process has been hypothesized to be a metabolic crisis,[3] where the muscle has been asked to stay tight for too long and the individual cells are running out of energy and start screaming out in pain. Research seems to hint at a close relationship between painful MFTPs and central sensitization.[4]

How to get rid of them?

Luckily, there are a few treatment options that work extremely well. Sadly, I've found both clinically and in my searches through the literature that massage, stretching, heat, therapeutic ultrasound, TENS, and light therapy[5] do

---

[3] Simons DG. New views of myofascial trigger points: etiology and diagnosis. *Arch Phys Med Rehabil.* 2008;89(1):157-159. doi:10.1016/j.apmr.2007.11.016

[4] Shah JP, Thaker N, Heimur J, Aredo JV, Sikdar S, Gerber L. Myofascial Trigger Points Then and Now: A Historical and Scientific Perspective. *PM R.* 2015;7(7):746-761. doi:10.1016/j.pmrj.2015.01.024

[5] Fagundes MG, Albuquerque JR dos S, Silva EJS, Dantas ACV, Lima TBW e. The effects of low-level laser in the treatment of myofascial pain syndrome:

                                             BRANDON RAMAKKO

not reliably resolve the issue (not that they don't provide some amount of relief). With experimentation, I found massage guns/machines work a bit better, but I find their results inconsistent person-to-person. **Ischemic compression, dry needling, and extracorporeal shockwave therapy** have all been shown to be reasonably effective.[6,7] If you need help, you may find chiropractors, massage therapists, acupuncturists, or physiotherapists who know one or more of these techniques.

I would argue that ischemic compression is the best with dry needling a close second. In fact, I find that each treatment works best for me with different muscles. Ischemic compression in particular has the advantage over needles because it can be done by anybody (even yourself or your partner), it is safe, and you can feel the muscle knot melting away so you have immediate feedback. Check out the treatments section of the book for more information on the techniques.

---

systematic review. *BrJP.* 2023;6(1):83-89. doi:10.5935/2595-0118.20230014-en

[6] Xu A, Huang Q, Rong J, Wu X, Deng M, Ji L. Effectiveness of ischemic compression on myofascial trigger points in relieving neck pain: A systematic review and meta-analysis. *J Back Musculoskelet Rehabil.* 2023;36(4):783-798. doi:10.3233/BMR-220045

[7] Zhang Q, Fu C, Huang L, et al. Efficacy of Extracorporeal Shockwave Therapy on Pain and Function in Myofascial Pain Syndrome of the Trapezius: A Systematic Review and Meta-Analysis. *Arch Phys Med Rehabil.* 2020;101(8):1437-1446. doi:10.1016/j.apmr.2020.02.013

DOES ARTHRITIS CAUSE PAIN?

To be clear, this section is talking about osteoarthritis (wear and tear) and not autoimmune arthritis (where the body's immune system is attacking itself). **Osteoarthritis**, the normal age-related changes to cartilage and bone, **has a poor correlation to pain**. There are a great number of people with arthritis diagnosable on X-ray with no pain. It may be a contributor to a cause of pain. It may cause pain in some. But there is strong evidence that, for a large percentage of people, arthritis results in no pain. In one study on hips in those aged 45-65, they found the prevalence of arthritis in those with hip pain was 13.3% and in those with no hip pain to be 9.5%. They concluded that diagnosing arthritis on X-ray has little use to determine the cause of pain since arthritis is so common in the asymptomatic (pain free).[8] You could infer from this study that maybe ⅓ of the time arthritis might be related to pain and that about 4% of the total hip pain was related to the arthritis. Describing arthritis as bone-on-bone grinding doesn't help those people with central sensitization and can make people fearful of exercising or being active resulting in all sorts of muscle and joint issues. Study after study finds that, statistically, pain scores and ability to function improves for people with arthritis

---

[8] Rondas GA, Macri EM, Oei EH, Bierma-Zeinstra SM, Rijkels-Otters HB, Runhaar J. Association between hip pain and radiographic hip osteoarthritis in primary care: the CHECK cohort. *Br J Gen Pract.* 2022;72(723):e722-e728. doi:10.3399/BJGP.2021.0547

when people do exercises/physiotherapy. The arthritis doesn't go away but they feel and perform better.[9,10] In one study involving squats (the exercise most people with knee pain avoid) they found there was significant improvement in pain relief, range of motion, muscle strength, and knee stability.[11] If anything, you can imagine using the knees more would make the arthritis worse… but, overall, the patients feel better. In my clinical opinion, unless there is a lot of swelling, bony chips in the joint locking it up, or bony growths at the edges large enough to limit the range of movement, arthritis is not an issue. If those conditions are met, then at that point, consider joint surgeries/replacements.

So, arthritis isn't necessarily painful. This type of thinking holds true for some other types of degenerative changes. Even degenerative rotator cuff tears in the shoulder might be pain free. If a radiologist sees a tear on the MRI, there is no guarantee the tear is actually painful.[12] One third of

------

[9] Golightly YM, Allen KD, Caine DJ. A comprehensive review of the effectiveness of different exercise programs for patients with osteoarthritis. *Phys Sportsmed.* 2012;40(4):52-65. doi:10.3810/psm.2012.11.1988

[10] Raposo, F., Ramos, M., & Lúcia Cruz, A. Effects of exercise on knee osteoarthritis: A systematic review. *Musculoskeletal Care.* 2021;19(4), 399–435. https://doi.org/10.1002/msc.1538

[11] Zhao Z, Wang R, Guo Y, et al. Static Low-Angle Squatting Reduces the Intra-Articular Inflammatory Cytokines and Improves the Performance of Patients with Knee Osteoarthritis. *Biomed Res Int.* 2019;2019:9617923. Published 2019, Oct 30. doi:10.1155/2019/9617923

[12] Minagawa H, Yamamoto N, Abe H, et al. Prevalence of symptomatic and asymptomatic rotator cuff tears in the general population: From mass-screening in one village. *J Orthop.* 2013;10(1):8-12. Published 2013, Feb 26. doi:10.1016/j.jor.2013.01.008

adults over the age of thirty with no back pain have a disc herniation on MRI.[13] Tendon tears can be painful and disc herniations can be painful, but they aren't necessarily painful, particularly if it is an older injury.

Imaging is great. We love to point to something structurally and say, "Look, there's the problem!" but a picture of a telephone doesn't tell you if it is ringing or not. Mild arthritis, disc degeneration, and disc bulges seen on imaging are very common findings and should not be worried about based on the image alone. People who are too worried about damage may develop a chronic pain disorder/central sensitization. Doctors and chiropractors can both be a source of chronic pain disorders. Some chiropractors X-ray every patient and, of course, every patient has disc degeneration and some arthritis.

"Look here, you are wearing out your back. If you don't want it to get worse, you have to come in for weekly chiropractic adjustments. We can keep the discs healthier."

The doctor might show you a disc herniation or arthritis and want to do something for you: that injection, that drug, and/or that surgical consult. Even if it isn't bad enough to result in a referral, the patient has this lasting image of damage in their mind which is not helpful.

---

[13] See the back section for more information.

DO CORTISONE/STEROID INJECTIONS HELP?

Injections for joint pain often contain cortisone (steroids) and sometimes lidocaine (anesthetic). These injections can help a great deal but should be used with caution. Medical doctors are ill equipped to help with musculoskeletal pain. All they have are injections, pills, and referrals. The optimist in me thinks that they are just trying to do anything they can with the tools they have. There is an overprescription problem with opioids, proton pump inhibitors, antidepressants, antibiotics, etc.[14,15] and similarly, injections are also overutilized. They can be given for problems where they cause more harm than good or injected in the wrong location. Even when appropriate, there may be better alternatives.

There is the assumption that the doctor knows where to inject or what structure is the painful one. Maybe cortisone is appropriate for acute inflammation of a bursa, but the pain could actually be from the tendon. Pain can be very tricky when it comes to its source. For example, a problem at T12

---

[14] Safer DJ. Overprescribed Medications for US Adults: Four Major Examples. *J Clin Med Res.* 2019;11(9):617-622. doi:10.14740/jocmr3906

[15] Heidelbaugh JJ, Kim AH, Chang R, Walker PC. Overutilization of proton-pump inhibitors: what the clinician needs to know. *Therap Adv Gastroenterol.* 2012;5(4):219-232. doi:10.1177/1756283X12437358

(bottom of the rib cage) can cause pain in the pelvis and hip. If they are injecting the sacroiliac joint (pelvis) or the hip joint then the injections (anesthetic and/or cortisone) are not going to help the problem. The relief should be within minutes for anesthetic and within hours for cortisone. I had a patient who hadn't received any relief for hip pain after receiving almost a dozen injections 2 days previous. Sounds to me like the injections were not in the correct location and that the doctor was using a shotgun approach to try to give her some relief. Cortisone may not be that good of a pain reliever anyway as it may be no better than placebo for back pain.[16]

If they can help sometimes, then what is the harm?

They can sometimes make problems much worse, both in terms of pain (after some initial relief), and by directly damaging tissues. Cortisone will thin cartilage, weaken tendons and ligaments, make skin thinner, and can even weaken bones. They increase the likelihood of tendon tears and increase the progression of arthritis.[17,18]

---

[16] Bogduk N. A narrative review of intra-articular corticosteroid injections for low back pain. *Pain Med.* 2005;6(4):287-296. doi:10.1111/j.1526-4637.2005.00048.x

[17] Brinks A, Koes BW, Volkers AC, Verhaar JA, Bierma-Zeinstra SM. Adverse effects of extra-articular corticosteroid injections: a systematic review. *BMC Musculoskelet Disord.* 2010;11:206. Published 2010 Sep 13. doi:10.1186/1471-2474-11-206

[18] Grillet B, Dequeker J. Intra-articular steroid injection. A risk-benefit assessment. *Drug Saf.* 1990;5(3):205-211. doi:10.2165/00002018-199005030-00005

When should cortisone injections be used?

Cortisone is a very strong anti-inflammatory and may act as a pain reliever. It will help a painful and swollen joint but it is uncalled for in just a painful joint. Unless the pain is too intense to move properly and/or do rehab, then there is an argument for cortisone for pain control to keep the joint mobile. If you already don't have cartilage in a joint and are waiting for knee replacement surgery, then it could be argued you should get the shot as there isn't any more cartilage to damage anyway (although it still might weaken the bone). You can actually take advantage of cortisone's destructive properties as it can be used to break up scar tissue or fibrous nodules. There are some particular pathologies like "trigger finger" where a single injection can resolve the issue entirely.[19] Ultrasound imaging guided injections can have better outcomes as the physician can make sure that the injection is going exactly where it needs to go.[20] I would not even consider an injection of cortisone without ultrasound guidance except in the most swollen of cases. For the temporary pain relief (although possibly more pain later) cortisone can be placed on top of a tendon but should never be injected into a tendon as cortisone damages tenocytes,

---

[19] Dala-Ali BM, Nakhdjevani A, Lloyd MA, Schreuder FB. The efficacy of steroid injection in the treatment of trigger finger. *Clin Orthop Surg.* 2012;4(4):263-268. doi:10.4055/cios.2012.4.4.263

[20] Sibbitt WL Jr, Kettwich LG, Band PA, et al. Does ultrasound guidance improve the outcomes of arthrocentesis and corticosteroid injection of the knee? . *Scand J Rheumatol.* 2012;41(1):66-72. doi:10.3109/03009742.2011.599071

the cells that maintain and heal tendons.[21] I've heard that when getting calcifications in a shoulder tendon aspirated (removed) that injecting a little cortisone into the bursa (fluid sac above the tendon) can prevent a red, swollen shoulder, which allows for faster recovery to normal daily activities. Even in this case, the cortisone is not required for recovery but for pain control. There is an issue with the progression of medical knowledge. Trochanteric bursitis, plantar fasciitis, lateral epicondylitis are common diagnoses for anyone with hip pain, foot pain, or elbow pain respectively and they all have "itis" in their name. The "itis" means inflammation. We **now** know that the majority of these patient's pain are due to a degenerative/deconditioning process rather than acute inflammation which means cortisone is uncalled for. These inflammatory diagnoses are mostly outdated but it may take decades for the healthcare community to adapt to this change.

There are other types of injections and options for the doctor aside from cortisone shots that will be covered later in the book such as: anesthetic injections/nerve blocks, PRP, prolotherapy, stem cells, or joint aspirations. In particular, anesthetics can let you identify the structure/region causing some of your pain if it provides relief, and a joint aspiration can provide relief from excess fluid by simply draining it.

---

[21] Spang C, Chen J, Backman LJ. The tenocyte phenotype of human primary tendon cells in vitro is reduced by glucocorticoids. *BMC Musculoskelet Disord.* 2016;17(1):467. Published 2016 Nov 10. doi:10.1186/s12891-016-1328-9

WHY IS NERVE PAIN SO STUBBORN?

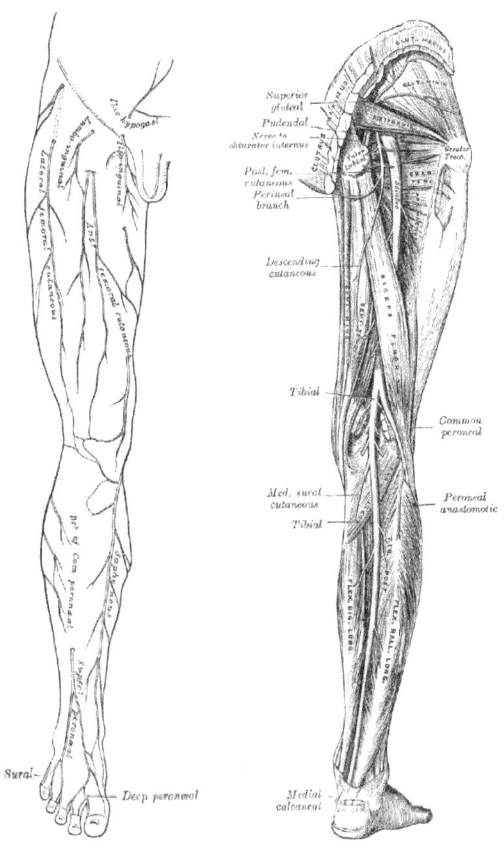

First off, many people think they have nerve pain that they don't. Secondly, people have multiple regions of nerve impingement/compression so that if you only treat one, the problem doesn't resolve entirely. Thirdly, nerve pain may be due to a structural issue that won't resolve without surgical intervention. Fourthly, significant nerve damage is very slow to heal. Fifthly, the nerve pain may have a systemic issue causing/contributing to it. For the sixth reason, refer to the earlier section about central sensitization!

If I had a nickel for every person that came in thinking they had sciatic nerve pain and it turned out to be muscle, fascia, and/or scar tissue, I could treat myself to a fancy steak dinner. Maybe 10% of the time, in my clinical experience, does it actually turn out to be a sciatic nerve issue. The interesting thing about the English language is that if a term is used incorrectly enough, the definition changes. Many definitions of "sciatica" now describe it as any pain going down the back of the leg. Sciatica could be pelvic joint pain, muscle pain, etc. Maybe the problem started as nerve pain but the chronic issue is now a combination of joint and muscle pain (muscle knots) with maybe a dash of central sensitization. Although I used "sciatica" as my example, this applies to nerve issues in the arms/hands as well.

Let's briefly talk about some terminology. A neuropathy is any problem with the nerve. A radiculopathy is a problem with the nerve root which is located where the nerve is separating from the spinal cord. Myelopathy is a problem with the spinal cord. Neuropathy and radiculopathy are more used when there is a loss of sensation or strength. Neuritis/radiculitis contains the "itis" for inflammation and is more specifically used when the nerve is painful but no losses otherwise. "Itis"-type nerve pain and muscle/joint pain can overlap and mimic each other.

There is something called double crush syndrome. In a double crush syndrome, the nerve is compressed at multiple locations. The effect on the nerve is more than additive. One unit of compression at two locations may be equivalent to 3 or 4 units of compression at just one location. These cases used to throw me for a loop when I naïvely began practicing. I would find one location with a problem, then treat it and watch the person get a bit better...but they wouldn't get 100% better: they would plateau. Now I know to check up and down the path of the nerve for all the places the nerve can be affected AND check all the joints and muscles that could mimic nerve pain referral.

Sometimes immediately after treatment, the patient's sensation and strength noticeably improves. With significant nerve compression over a long period of time, or if there is chemical damage (chemotherapy), the nerve may take a long time to heal (if it ever does). It may take months before significant improvement in sensation and/or strength. One example case was of someone who may have been drugged while out drinking because she swears she only had two drinks. This hypermobile individual woke up with her arm in a partially dislocated position. When she uncontorted herself, she could only move some of her muscles. Other muscles were "dead." Significant compression overnight was all it took to cause enough nerve damage (from lack of nutrients) to significantly damage the nerve. It was months of work before her arm was relatively normal again. Interestingly, this type of arm paresis is associated with drinking and is called "Saturday night palsy" and can happen by passing out with your arm over the back of a chair.

It would be remiss of me to not mention that nutritional deficiencies, cancer, and diseases can also cause nerve symptoms. A B12 deficiency, diabetes, alcoholism, etc. can all cause nerve symptoms in arms and legs. Cancerous tumors can directly compress nerves, or cancer treatment can cause nerve damage. Chemotherapy involves injecting the patient with poison, hoping it kills the cancer before it kills the patient. Sixty percent of chemotherapy patients experience neuropathy (nerve problems), but luckily 6 months later that number decreases to 30%.[22]

---

[22] Seretny M, Currie GL, Sena ES, et al. Incidence, prevalence, and predictors of chemotherapy-induced peripheral neuropathy: A systematic review and meta-analysis. *Pain.* 2014;155(12):2461-2470. doi:10.1016/j.pain.2014.09.020

A NOTE ABOUT SYSTEMIC DISEASES AND NUTRITION

This book is not about problems involving the systems of the body, but these problems can mimic the typical chronic neuromusculoskeletal problems discussed in this book. In those individuals, if you only address one issue, then it may appear like the problem is not resolving.

Blood tests and imaging can help rule in or out autoimmune disorders where the body is attacking itself. Some of these conditions are Lupus, rheumatoid arthritis, Crohn's, etc. There are many such conditions. These conditions often involve the whole body but may start in just one region. For example, psoriatic arthritis can affect just one finger (but likely both hands).

I would include hormones in a list of systemic issues. We are all familiar with the havoc menopause or the menstrual cycle can have on a woman's body. Mental state, lifestyle, and nutrition each play a role in the levels of the hormones as well. Tumors, cancerous or otherwise, can affect the hormones if the tumor is in a hormone producing organ like the thyroid. Diabetes can also be considered a hormone issue and the symptoms can cause blindness, burning thigh pain, numbness/tingling in hands, etc.

Nutrition, or more specifically the lack of nutrition, can lead to or exacerbate medical problems. A zinc deficiency can double the healing time of an ankle sprain. A vitamin B12 deficiency can cause nerve symptoms (tingling, numbness). In general, taking more than you need of a vitamin does not help. If there is a deficiency, it can help a great deal. You can't always go by the daily recommended values either, as some individuals may require more. I sometimes have specific recommendations, but I normally recommend a good multivitamin, omega-3 supplement, and a vitamin D supplement.

Not only do you need to get enough nutrition, but you may need to avoid excess of some things, like sugar, or something your body is intolerant to. Sometimes food itself can be in excess as in high blood pressure or obesity. Type-II diabetes stems from too much sugar (some people don't know that type-II diabetes is reversible in the early stages). Gout can result in painful joints and stems from too much alcohol and rich foods. Smoking can slow healing and increase the risk of musculoskeletal injuries.

If you have chronic problems, don't neglect this stuff. I was told I have arthritis in my hands and feet in my early twenties. I had daily hand and foot pain but experimenting with diet and supplements eventually resulted in greatly reducing that pain and eliminated the need for prescription anti-inflammatories.

COULD THE PAIN BE FROM CANCER OR AN INTERNAL ORGAN?

While the focus of the book is musculoskeletal pain and I am trying to keep the book positive, it is inevitable that I should mention cancer and organ pain. While the treatments to cancer can cause serious side effects (nerve damage in particular for chemotherapy), I'm writing this chapter in reference to the cancerous tumors and metastasis.

Some tumors in bones are benign in that they won't spread or kill you but they can grow and become painful and troublesome like giant cell tumors and aneurysmal bone cysts. Both of which cause the bone to physically become larger and weaker. Many types of cancer metastasize (spread) to the spine such as lung, prostate, breast, multiple myeloma, and more. This can result in progressively worsening back pain. The tumors can compress the nerves leading to worsening nerve symptoms (loss of sensation, tingling, and muscle weakness). The key here is progressively worsening. Cancer pain does not respond well to muscle treatments and exercises. Throughout this book, I encourage you to seek out professional help and to try different practitioners and different treatments, to find all the problems and try all the treatments to get you as good as you can be. If you are continuing to worsen over months/years, particularly if you have increased risk factors: over fifty years of age, history of cancer (personal and/or family), and/or are a smoker, then consider having a doctor send you for a bone scan, PET scan, MRI, CT, or X-ray. Bone scans and PET scans can detect cancer anywhere in the body. The more active the cancer, the brighter it will be on imaging.

Organs don't typically have a lot of pain receptors in them. At least, not in the same way your skin does. It would be a waste of resources as your organs don't interact with the outside world. Organ damage/pain can be interpreted by the nervous system as coming from nearby muscles and joints. This organ-type pain may be from an infection, cancerous tumor, or dysfunction. Since lots of internal organs are associated with food digestion, if the pain is related to your eating habits (example, if it always occurs 20 minutes after eating) then that is one hint. If it doesn't respond to muscle treatments, that is another. Sometimes the pain is dependent on body positioning: standing versus lying on your back. Kidney pain is often felt in the back on one side (look for pain with urination or discolored urine). Pancreas pain refers to the central or center-left mid-low back (look for jaundice and fecal changes). Stomach pain can refer to mid back in the lower ribcage. This is just a sampling of organ referred pain. The body, interpreting organ pain from an area, can stiffen the muscles there. Also, muscle and joint aches are common. It is possible that you have normal aches combined with something internal. For example, you get some relief from muscle work/exercises, but never full relief. Keep in mind, a good therapist will be re-evaluating regularly and changing the treatment plan to ensure continued improvements over time (although sometimes 2 steps forward, one step back). In cases where improvement seems to plateau, think about the other systems in your body as it may be prudent to get full blood work done and/or urine testing.

DO I NEED TO SEE A THERAPIST REGULARLY?

I often get asked if regular physiotherapy, chiropractor, acupuncture, and/or massage visits are necessary. Ideally, no. A good, ethical, physiotherapist or chiropractor should be trying to get you to the point that you never need more care. Most people can achieve this, but it can sometimes take a lot of dedication on the part of the patient and the health practitioner.

Sadly, common business practices and/or laziness means they may not be making your long-term success their priority. If you continue to have bad habits, then your tissues will be under increased strain. Regular visits to receive passive treatment (treatment the therapist/physician does to you) may help keep the pain at bay. Lack of rehab (poor muscle control) can predispose people to continuously reinjure themselves, requiring frequent visits for care. The therapist should be constantly re-evaluating your state, modifying the treatments, ensuring continued progression, checking for and eliminating bad habits, and instilling good habits and lifestyle changes.

Some people may benefit from semi-regular visits to check on things and to point out any exercises or changes the patient might do to maximize their quality of life. Individuals going through tough times might benefit from regular support for muscle pains while going through a phase that might not allow for exercises, proper ergonomics, stretching breaks, proper nutrition, etc. Individuals that have a significant asymmetry such as one leg being a couple inches longer than the other or someone who must use a single crutch will be prone to returning muscle aches.

BAD POSTURE AND OTHER BAD HABITS

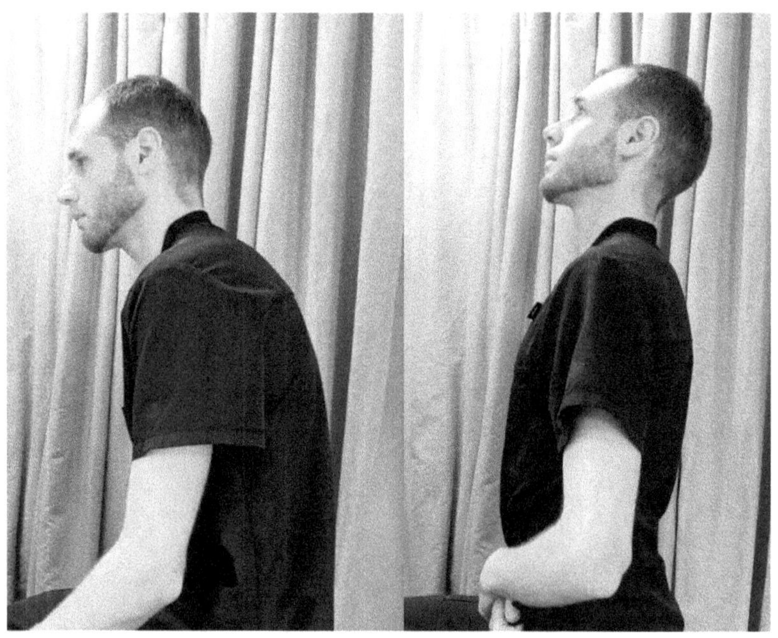

Bad posture doesn't directly cause pain… unless it is held for long periods of time. A healthy individual can slump for 15 minutes and be fine. Bad posture increases the force on ligaments and muscles. This isn't beyond what these tissues are normally capable of handling (short term) but if you combine bad posture with long periods of time, this is where problems start.

Bad posture is a bad habit.

Sometimes this habit is hard to break as sitting with proper posture after years of not doing it may be painful. Sometimes muscle and joint work is necessary for the individual to feel comfortable sitting comfortably so they can work on the good habit of good posture. We can extend the discussion in this section to other bad habits involving the body. If someone injures their ankle/foot, they may walk with a limp until healed. Part of this limp may persist since it has become a habit and can contribute to hip, knee, or foot pain. These bad habits may have to be fixed to stay pain free.

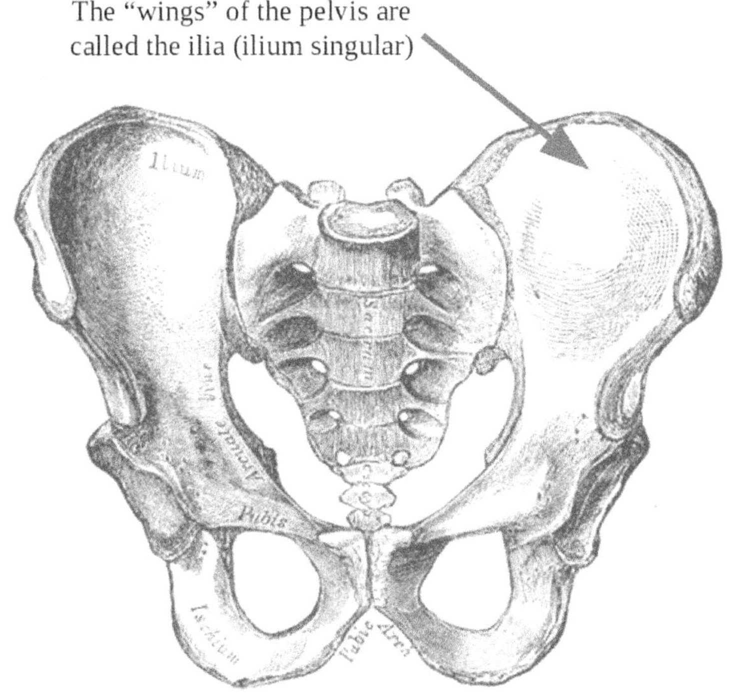

How to fix bad posture?

The exact fix to bad posture can vary a bit person-to-person, but I'll include a bit here to get you started with seated posture.

First, let us start with the position of the pelvis. There should be a gentle inward curve of your low back when you are seated. That is what all those lumbar supports are supposed to help you with. Even if sitting unsupported, you should naturally sit with this curvature. To find this ideal curvature, I normally start with pelvic tilts (tilting the pelvis too far forward and too far back). Notice how your height changes as you move the pelvis (I find physically grabbing the wings/ilia of the pelvis helps with this). When you have your pelvis tilted back, you are short and as you move forward you get taller and taller until you reach maximum height at which point is sort of plateaus. That first peak is the point where your back is the happiest and is called "neutral pelvis." All the vertebrae are neatly stacked on top of each other and your muscles are doing the least work. If this position hurts and feels like something is too tight, then seek help to stretch something or work out the pain. If it just feels different, then make it your new habit! This is a relatively easy habit to get used to if you make a concerted effort for a week.

Already you should be sitting much taller with your pelvis in the correct position. Now you just need to hold your shoulders back, right? WRONG. Well, you can try, but you are not likely to be successful in this. Your posture muscles aren't normally controlled by the conscious brain. Whether your shoulders are being pulled back or not is left up to your subconscious once you start focusing on something else. How to trick your subconscious into using the muscles that pull your shoulder blades back and down? Why not a quick muscle warmup multiple times a day? Most of my patients have had success with this strategy. The exact exercise doesn't matter as long as you like it, it's effective, and it feels good as you need to do it multiple times a day. I'll place a sample exercise at the end of this section. Maybe once an hour with an office job. I recommend 80% effort of the muscles that act to bring the shoulders down and back for 5 to 6 second holds, 3 repetitions: Bruegger's relief position, wide rows, wall angels, close rows, pull downs, arm windmills, bow and arrow, etc. You should notice afterward that the muscles above your shoulders feel lighter (see "muscle energy techniques" for an explanation) and your shoulders are naturally sitting a bit further back. If your pecs are particularly tight, then stretching them beforehand may be beneficial.

Here are instructions for Brugger's relief position:

- Sit up tall as if you are being pulled up by a thread attached to the top of your head. Chin is tucked slightly.

- Make sure your pelvis is tilted such that you have a gentle inward curve in your low back (neutral pelvis).

- Pull your shoulder blades down.

- Rotate your arms outwards. Make sure you aren't overextending your back. You may have to lightly engage your abdominals.

- Hold for 5-20 seconds. Repeat if necessary.

- Repeat the procedure as needed throughout the day such as every hour of office work.

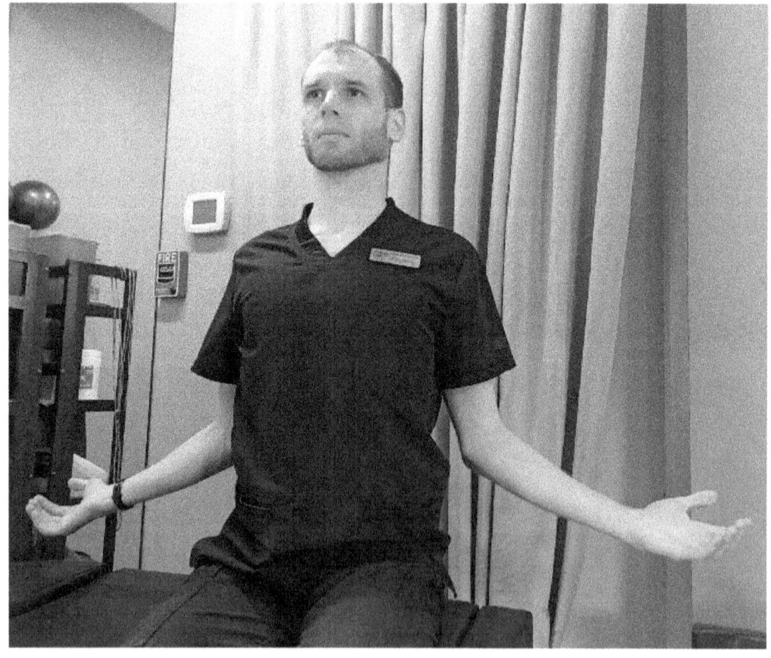

If you feel particularly stuck with your upper back rounded forward, you can try a lengthy passive stretch of the upper back. Just like a gymnast stretches their leg muscles for minutes instead of seconds to achieve their splits, stretching the back for lengthier periods of time can be more helpful than a quick stretch. You can bend over the back of a chair, armrest, etc. or lie on a pillow or bunched up towel under your upper back, between your shoulder blades. A deep breath out can further accentuate the stretch. Hold for 30 seconds to 5 minutes.

The neck is a bit trickier. Some individuals need a whole exercise program to help with the neck. The most typical posture exercise involves bringing the head back while tucking the chin. One variation of this is I have patients try is to have them push the back of their head against a wall while keeping the chin tucked. They could also use the headrest of their car (what else are you going to do while stuck at a red light?). Five to ten second holds for a few repetitions. Having the correct screen height can help greatly for neck posture. The top of the monitor should be at eye level or higher. Once the neck is moving better, use it or lose it. Try to use the entire range of motion of your neck every day. Make a habit of looking up and/or tilting your head side to side when you stretch or get up from a working session.

DO I NEED AN ERGONOMICS ASSESSMENT?

Our work space can play a huge role in our day-to-day comfort. Taking frequent breaks and using standing desks, exercise balls, lumbar supports, foot rests, monitor stands, special computer mice, etc., can all be beneficial. Even if you have had an ergonomic assessment done and have the best equipment, make sure these things are working for you in the long run. Arm rests can be beneficial but, particularly if they are too low, you might slump to reach them (I removed my armrests because they were causing me to slump). A common recommendation is to have the top of the monitor at eye level, but I find I still slumped, so that where I tended to look (center screen) was at eye level. So, I normally recommend the monitor an inch or two above eye level. Exercise balls make for a great workout while sitting but will tire you out fast. They are best used to break up monotonous sitting during a break or as a temporary chair for 10-30 minutes. We have a tendency to like things within arm's reach. Having a monitor stand so you can bring the monitor, not just to the correct level, but closer to you can help. Keeping the hand pronated (palm down) for hours can cause or aggravate "carpal tunnel"-like symptoms. Taking breaks to work out the pronator teres (see the elbow section), or having a mouse which doesn't require your hand to be fully rotated can be beneficial. Switching the main mouse button on a normal mouse can have the effect of using it differently with slightly less pronation. If you use the back of the seat while working, having a lumbar support can be helpful to maintain the proper curvature in your low back. Note that even if you are sitting with perfect form, because we are not designed to sit for hours on end, you will still feel fatigue and discomfort eventually.

ARE SUPPORT BRACES HELPFUL?

Braces are sometimes a necessary part of protecting a freshly injured joint while still allowing the individual to move around. With a fresh ankle or knee sprain, you don't want to accidentally re-injure the ligament while it is healing.

Braces and crutches can alter how your body moves. In fact, a large portion of rehab is sometimes getting rid of bad habits from protecting a joint or only using one side of the body. Using muscles incorrectly can lead to those nasty muscle knots, knee/joint clicking, and increases the likelihood of injury. Not using muscles can lead to tendon and muscle deconditioning/weakening.

For chronic issues, I try to get people away from reliance on braces and supports as much as possible. If you don't have a fresh injury that needs protection then **reliance on braces can be a contributing factor in the continued persistence of your chronic pain syndrome**.

Specifically, let's talk about neck and back braces. These braces are so common that you can find them at grocery stores. Neck braces are only for structural instability and/or unstable neck fractures but some wear one whenever their neck "goes out." Lumbar (low back) braces are uncalled for unless you are trying to set a world record in weightlifting. Using either will further worsen proper muscle control perpetuating and worsening your condition.

Posture braces that force you into position don't work as well as posture devices that just remind you to maintain good posture. You don't want a strap that holds you in place, you want to train your muscles to do it. Kinesiotape might be a good in-between that feels supportive but doesn't interfere with your muscles doing their job.

What about heel lifts?

About 90% of people have one leg a bit longer than the other with the average being about 5mm.[23] It might be logical to try to correct this with a small wedge, called a heel lift, or custom footwear to compensate for the shorter leg. While there is a subset of people who have been helped using this strategy, our bodies are already so great at adapting that many don't benefit from a heel lift. Problems normally only correlate to differences greater than 2cm. You have lived your whole life adapting to the difference so sometimes people get worse with heel lifts or, once used to the heel lifts, they feel uncomfortable walking barefoot or in flip-flops. It is a tool to consider but I try to help the ankle, knee, hip, pelvis, and back issues through other means first before trying this method. Double heel lifts or wedge shoes may

---

[23] Knutson GA. Anatomic and functional leg-length inequality: a review and recommendation for clinical decision-making. Part I, anatomic leg-length inequality: prevalence, magnitude, effects and clinical significance. *Chiropr Osteopat.* 2005;13:11. Published 2005, Jul 20. doi:10.1186/1746-1340-13-11

help with Achilles (posterior ankle) tendon pain during the recovery process.[24]

What about orthotics?

Orthotics are a big business (more than 3 billion USD).[25] I have seen making changes in footwear (orthotics or particular style of shoe) result in a huge difference to someone's recovery and/or preventing pain from reoccurring. That being said, some people have not responded well to changes in footwear, and changing footwear alone is often not sufficient for long-standing pain. Just like with other supports, too much support can impede the body's natural functioning: consider that our feet evolved for walking without any support.

Is it my bed? Do I need a special pillow?

Maybe, but don't necessarily go out right now to buy the most expensive option. There have been many pillow studies (mostly of low quality) and many (but not all) found no

---

[24] Rabusin CL, Menz HB, McClelland JA, et al. Efficacy of heel lifts versus calf muscle eccentric exercise for mid-portion Achilles tendinopathy (HEALTHY): a randomised trial. *Br J Sports Med.* 2021;55(9):486-492. doi:10.1136/bjsports-2019-101776

[25] https://www.fortunebusinessinsights.com/industry-reports/foot-orthotic-insoles-market-100348

correlation between symptoms and pillow types.[26,27] I delved into the data of one study and there were subsets within each group that got better and some who got worse. This tells me that personal experimentation is in order. Every patient is a unique snowflake and you have to find what works for you. Typically, I recommend smaller, thinner pillows, for back sleepers. I recommend experimenting with a rolled-up hand towel to see if you like a little support under the neck. Sometimes placing a smushed up hand towel between the shoulder blades or taking your pillow and having it just under the shoulder can also encourage a more neutral posture for sleeping. Side sleepers often do better with double pillows so their neck isn't tilted while sleeping. I don't recommend belly sleeping. I do recommend a wedge under the legs (back sleeping) for back pain or a pillow between the legs (on side) for hip pain. I find that the back and hip suggestions often aren't needed in most with sufficient back and hip treatment/rehab. In particular, the hip requirement is often gone in a treatment or two of those pesky muscle knots! Back issues are sometimes helped by working on the iliacus/psoas muscles and the SI joints.

---

[26] Gordon SJ, Grimmer KA, Buttner P. Pillow preferences of people with neck pain and known spinal degeneration: a pilot randomized controlled trial. *Eur J Phys Rehabil Med.* 2019;55(6):783-791. doi:10.23736/S1973-9087.19.05263-8

[27] Shields N, Capper J, Polak T, Taylor N. Are cervical pillows effective in reducing neck pain? *New Zealand Journal of Physiotherapy* 2006; 34(1): 3-9. https://www.ncbi.nlm.nih.gov/books/NBK73379/

IS IT BECAUSE OF MY WEAK CORE?

I recently attended a conference where the physiotherapist Dr. Bohdanna Zozulak (author of *Master Your Core*) gave a talk where she was sharing some of her research on the relationship between the core and injury prevention. This research involved testing proprioception rather than the usual studies that connect core endurance with pain or injury. The research points to the importance of intersegmental control to react in an instant to stabilize what needs to be stabilized. Poor proprioception (sense of where the joint is and what it is doing) increased the likelihood of women injuring their knee by 2-3 times on average.[28] She said that retraining the core is more like learning a language than an exercise. Neuromuscular re-education requires variety: expanding the repertoire of what your body can do, discovering what it has trouble with and practicing until it is perfect, and then moving on to the next movement or a more demanding version of the same movement.

You can imagine that those people with better core endurance might also have better core proprioception because in

---

[28] Zazulak BT, Hewett TE, Reeves NP, Goldberg B, Cholewicki J. The effects of core proprioception on knee injury: a prospective biomechanical-epidemiological study. *Am J Sports Med.* 2007;35(3):368-373. doi:10.1177/0363546506297909

　　　　　　　　　　　　　BRANDON RAMAKKO

all likelihood they haven't been injured, did proper rehab, and/or are more active. Most core research has been using endurance and strength tests, but I think they are learning the wrong lessons. If it was just about endurance and strength why would Tai Chi be so effective for back pain, even when compared with core workouts?[29,30] If you think about it, Tai Chi (or T'ai Chi) is just slow controlled bending, twisting, and weight shifting motions and, logically, improves neuromuscular control. Tai Chi definitely isn't what people would consider a "core workout."

My takeaway from this is that the core is important, but a balanced, well controlled, core is more important than pure endurance and strength one for injury prevention and for those in chronic pain. A million crunches and holding a plank for an hour shouldn't be the goal, but being able to confidently move your body in a controlled fashion and your core being able to react at a moment's notice should be. (Adding in some endurance and strength exercises wouldn't hurt... Maybe it is time to get that six pack.)

---

[29] Zou L, Zhang Y, Liu Y, et al. The Effects of Tai Chi Chuan Versus Core Stability Training on Lower-Limb Neuromuscular Function in Aging Individuals with Non-Specific Chronic Lower Back Pain. *Medicina (Kaunas)*. 2019;55(3):60. Published 2019 Mar 3. doi:10.3390/medicina55030060

[30] Wang X-Q, Xiong H-Y, Du S-H, Yang Q-H and Hu L (2022) The effect and mechanism of traditional Chinese exercise for chronic low back pain in middle-aged and elderly patients: A systematic review. *Front. Aging Neurosci.* 14:935925. doi: 10.3389/fnagi.2022.935925

HOW TO EXERCISE/REHAB PROPERLY?

A body builder, a gymnast, a rock climber, and a chronic neck pain patient—each needs different types of exercise. Each person has a different goal: making muscles as large as possible, increasing muscle power, improving strength/endurance, and neuromuscular retraining. In this section, I'm not going to be going over specific exercise programs but an overview of types of exercises and general strategies. Maybe you can use these strategies to modify what you already do to maximize the benefit you are after.

How to build muscles efficiently?

We have to overuse those muscles. You have to create microtears in those muscles. The body's response to this is going to be to build the muscle bigger and stronger. In general, you want to be pushing your body to the limit with a small number of repetitions with as much weight/resistance as you can. How many reps exactly? Roughly 5-20. I often tell people, "until failure." Until you lose form or you physically can't anymore. Even then, you could switch to a lighter weight and continue until even that is too much. You should do at least 2 sets, if not more. When it comes to muscle building, any exercise worth doing is worth doing twice.

And what about afterwards? You need to give your body the building blocks necessary to rebuild those muscles and you have to give the body time for the repairs. I recommend supplementing your diet with protein shakes when working out like this. You also can't work out your muscles like this every day. You have to wait until the muscles fully heal, this is why people have "leg day", "arm day", etc. You can work out every day if, each time you work out, you always work a different region. Give each region about 1-2 days to recover. Each region can be worked 2-3 times a week.

Don't use age as an excuse. The combination of increased protein intake and resistance exercises (weights, body weight, and/or resistance bands) has been found to increase muscle mass in even those 65+.[31]

How to retrain muscle control?

If your leg or arm was in a cast, if you have been bedridden for a week or more, or you have been limping from an ankle injury, then you have spent a week or more not using your muscles properly. The control and coordination might be off. Some muscles might already be weak and some muscles might be tighter. If muscles have been inactive long enough, the muscles have atrophied (wasted away) and tendons can become weakened and tender (tendinosis). You might have to rebuild muscle strength, recondition tendons, break up scar tissue, stretch tight muscles, and work out muscle

---

[31] Voulgaridou G, Papadopoulou SD, Spanoudaki M, et al. Increasing Muscle Mass in Elders through Diet and Exercise: A Literature Review of Recent RCTs. *Foods*. 2023;12(6):1218. Published 2023 Mar 13. doi:10.3390/foods12061218

knots (with ischemic compression) concurrently with, or even before, starting to retrain muscle control and coordination.

I like to compare retraining muscles to learning to play an instrument. You don't just learn one note and stop after that. You would get better at playing that one note, but once mastered, practicing it more won't make you a better musician. You have to learn new notes, you have to learn more challenging songs—it has to be challenging. You can, and should, practice often (daily) to learn an instrument in a timely manner. Now take this idea to brain-muscle retraining.

So, frequent, mentally challenging exercises are needed for those needing retraining: someone coming out of a coma might need to relearn to walk, the individual just recovered from an ankle sprain may need to relearn how to control the ankle and maybe needs to relearn how to toe-off (push-off) properly when walking. Someone after a back injury may have to relearn to use the muscles in bending forward. Someone after a "crick in the neck" (torticollis) may need to relearn fine motor control of the neck, etc. You don't need to take rest days like a bodybuilder might because you aren't pushing your muscles physically past their limits, you are working your brain instead.

So far, this all sounds like proper recovery from an acute injury, and this is a book about chronic pain, so how is this relevant? **Not rehabbing properly can lead to chronic pain, and rehab can be the path out of chronic pain.**

The exercises should be challenging. By "challenging," I don't mean the amount of weight/resistance. I'm referring to mentally challenging to perform perfectly. Correct form and smoothness are more important than weight/power/speed. If the exercise is too easy, it isn't worth doing. Let's take balance for example. You might start off balancing on one foot with eyes open, then balancing while shifting a weight from your left to right hand, then balancing eyes closed, then balancing on a balance board (unstable surface), etc. With rehabbing the neck, I often explore their range of motion slowly. If their neck jitters with a certain motion, then that becomes their homework. Once that motion is smooth, they should explore other motions (X, circle, etc.) until they find another motion that is challenging and practice that. Eventually the neck can do any motion perfectly!

What about muscles that need improved control **and** strength?

This is where it gets tricky… but not as tricky as you might think. If you lean towards neuromuscular training with frequent, gentle but challenging, slow exercise, or you go full muscle building with high intensity, multiple set exercises every few days, both groups seem to get some improvement. It is condition and person specific about which one you should lean more heavily towards. I err on the side of control first. If your control is so bad that working out causes your muscles to spasm/tighten, then you have to start with control.

You can also aim right between the two and do exercises every day, but if you do so much that you are sore the next day, you can just take a "rest day" or limit the more physically strenuous exercises every second day.

How to warm up for exercise to prevent injury?

To prevent injury, you want to prepare your body for the exercise. This doesn't just mean the muscles warmed up or getting your heartrate up. Your brain's control of the body should also be warmed up. Prepare the brain for what it can expect. A weightlifting routine could be prepared for by running through similar motions with no weight or less weights as an example. You can even go beyond the exercises range of motion to prepare the brain for control of the joint if things go beyond your expectations.

Should you stretch before exercise?

You shouldn't do lengthy passive stretching before exercising in general. You should actively (using your muscles) run your joints through their ranges of motion which prepares your body to use and coordinate those muscles/joints throughout that range. Long passive stretches can be done after exercise. There is an exception to this rule. If you are going to be doing neuromuscular re-education exercises (slow, controlled movements) there can be a benefit to stretching before exercises if your motion is limited. You may want to train your brain-body coordination using your full range of motion.

Is stretching more important than exercises?

                    BRANDON RAMAKKO

Stretching doesn't have the health benefits of other forms of physical activity: it doesn't improve heart health, reduce diabetes risk, improve lean body mass, improve balance, improve muscle coordination, improve strength, etc.[32] As discussed in other locations in this book, chronically tight muscles only temporarily benefit from stretches. If your brain wants the muscles to spasm tight, then they might tighten up again within an hour of being stretched/relaxed. In such circumstances, focusing on rehab and control-type exercises is a better use of time.

Stretching may take priority if you notice an asymmetry in flexibility/movement and/or your mobility is limited. If you can't do an exercise properly or symmetrically you are better off focusing on improving flexibility. Stretching post workout can prevent loss of range of motion. Some stretching just prior to neuromuscular training exercises may be useful.

Should stretching be painful?

 NO!!! Stretching should not be painful. If it is, then treatment of muscle knots, scar tissue, or fascial adhesion may be necessary. You shouldn't force stretches to the point of pain because you can tear stuff, ultimately reducing your flexibility.

---

[32] Physical activity guidelines by the American government department of health and human services: https://health.gov/sites/default/files/2019-09/Physical_Activity_Guidelines_2nd_edition.pdf

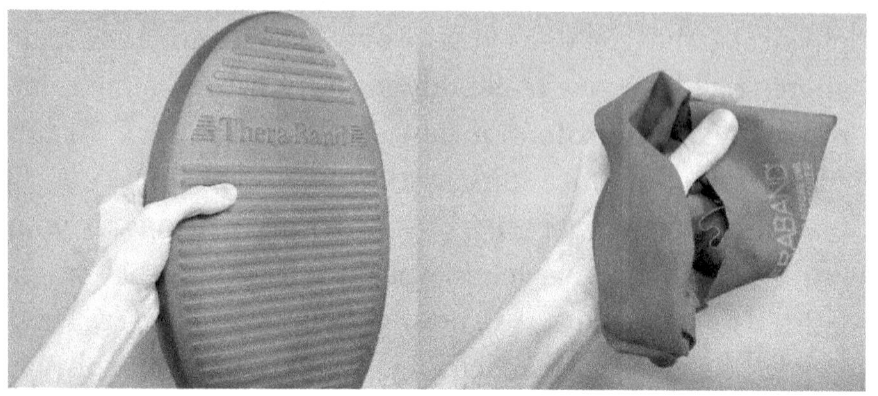

Do I need expensive equipment?

If the focus is on rehabilitation, control, maintenance, and functional movements, you don't need to involve heavy weights and expensive equipment, but everyone's goals or problems might be different. Body weight is typically sufficient. A couple light weights (2-12 lbs. or even soup cans may work) and/or TheraBands might be useful for shoulder exercises. A wobble/balance board may be useful for balance training and/or ankle rehab (I recommend the half circles more than dome for rehab). The balance pads are awesome as cushions for your knees for any hip passive stretch that involves putting your knee on the floor. TheraBands are great for hip, knee, and ankle rehab. An exercise ball is amazing for strengthening the larger core muscles. (You will never do crunches on the floor again after using an exercise ball.)

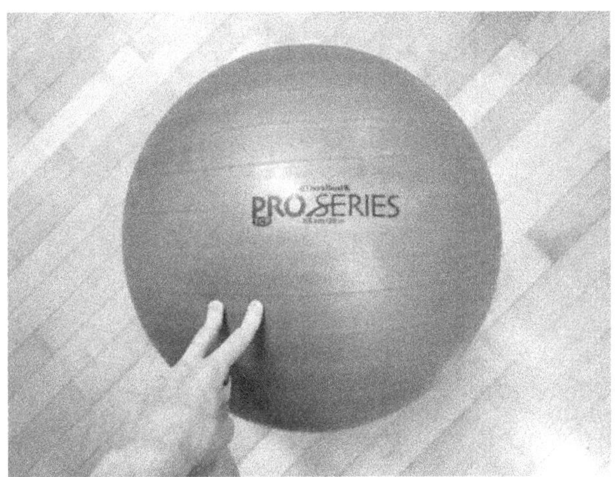

What to do once better?

Keep your body active as much as possible and expose your body to a variety of motions so it doesn't forget. Throwing in your rehab exercises, every once in a while, is one strategy. I've been using a quest 3 VR headset which is both fun and better than playing a sedentary game. Swimming and floating around in the water is great. Playing games with the kids or grandkids is fun and rewarding... don't just sit in a chair. Get up and play ball with them and chase them around.

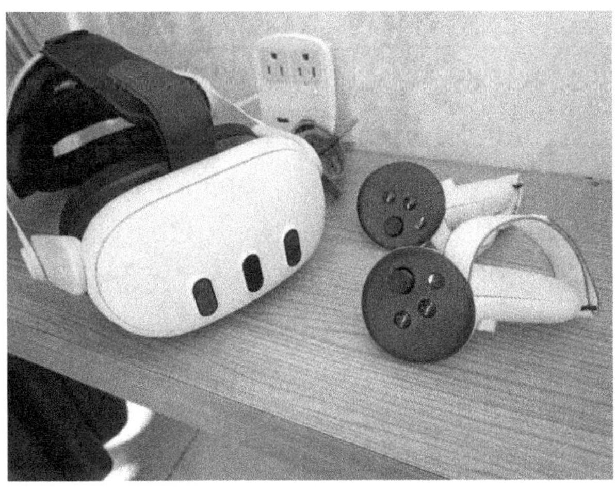

CHRONIC TENDON PAIN (Tendinosis)

Tendons are the connection between the muscles and the bones. They can be injured/torn and/or they can become swollen, tender, and weakened. Any issue with a tendon can be called a tendinopathy, but that isn't very specific. An "-itis" is inflammatory, so an acute, sudden, inflammation of a tendon is a tendinitis. This term is outdated and has been improperly overused. There is no such thing as chronic tendinitis. While inflammatory markers might be elevated, the cellular cause of the issue is not inflammatory. If it is swollen from an acute/sudden tear, then "tear" is the more appropriate diagnosis (sometimes requires ultrasound imaging for confirmation). Degenerative conditions have an "-osis" to them, and so a degenerated, deconditioned, swollen, tender, and weakened tendon is a tendinosis. A tendinosis is often misdiagnosed as a chronic tendinitis. Tendinosis is a chronic problem which develops over weeks to months. Tendinosis results from a mismatch of wear and tear and regular upkeep. Our body is constantly rebuilding and maintaining our tissues, and if the upkeep isn't keeping up with the wear and tear, then you get a tendinosis. Either you are overusing that tendon and/or the upkeep is below the required level. If you haven't been pushing your body to its limits, it may have decided to stop investing so many resources into maintaining the strength of the tendon. It is sometimes the "use it or lose it." You are so inactive that your tendons weaken. Inactivity can also mess with your muscle coordination, possibly increasing the wear on the tendons. Note that Gout can mimic or aggravate tendon pain/problems too. Tendinosis can be diagnosed via MRI and ultrasound but a tender tendon that is aggravated by overuse is almost always a tendinosis. Muscle knot pain can mimic a tendinosis, though, as the muscle pain can refer to the tendon location.

How to treat tendinosis?

There are a few strategies to fix tendons. Some are more extreme than others. One treatment is fenestration. Fenestration means to poke holes through something. Since the body isn't strengthening the tendon on its own, the doctor purposefully pokes a whole bunch of holes/tears in the tendon (with anesthesia). Now the tendon is very damaged and the body has to fix it. You hope it fixes it to be stronger and healthier. Similarly, PRP or dextrose injections may both help as they can encourage healing. Avoid cortisone injections, as this will weaken the tendon further, even if it does provide some short-term relief. Red light therapy and/or extracorporeal shockwave therapy might be useful. Exercises are the most common and consistently effective form of treatment.[33]

---

[33] Irby A, Gutierrez J, Chamberlin C, Thomas SJ, Rosen AB. Clinical management of tendinopathy: A systematic review of systematic reviews evaluating the effectiveness of tendinopathy treatments. *Scand J Med Sci Sports.* 2020;30(10):1810-1826. doi:10.1111/sms.13734

The tenocytes, the cells that repair the tendon, can be activated with high amounts of tension on the tendon so exercises that load the tendon in tension can kick start the rebuilding process. This can be a little tricky. I've heard multiple stories of physiotherapists pushing people too far and the tendon rupturing/tearing completely. These are weakened tendons that might have tears in them, so you have to ramp up the tension slowly throughout the rehab process. Pain for these types of exercises may be present but shouldn't exceed a 3/10 on the pain scale. A physiotherapist or chiropractor who uses ultrasound imaging can be useful in these cases to visually monitor the state of the tendon but that isn't usually required. The exercises are normally eccentric (with the muscle lengthening) as your muscles are strongest during these types of exercises. See the ankle section of this book for an example exercise for the Achilles tendon.

What about a bursitis?

Bursas are cushions between the tendons and other structures. These bursas are very thin, fluid-filled sacs. A "bursitis" is inflammation/swelling of the bursa which is normally an acute issue (sudden and short lasting), rather than a chronic problem. Many people seem to be diagnosed with chronic "bursitis." It used to be a common diagnosis with hip and shoulder pain. We now know that these bursas, even when they have extra fluid in them, are rarely the cause of pain (particularly for the hip). The extra fluid in the bursa can be related to the real cause of the chronic pain/problem which typically involves a tendon injury. A true, acute, inflammatory bursitis is one of the rare cases that cortisone injections are appropriate. Sadly, since the diagnosis has been overused over the years, needless cortisone shots are common. Changes in healthcare are slow. The updated information takes time to make its way to working health professionals who might finish their medical practicing career without ever having corrected their thinking about bursitis and cortisone.

SCAR TISSUE/FASCIAL PAIN

The fascia is the layer of tissue separating one structure from another. I like to think about it as everything inside you is wrapped in plastic bags. If there has been an injury, the plastic bags can get stuck together in the healing process. They can also get stuck together with lack of movement. This feels like a sharp pulling pain or a pinch. Sometimes there is no pain, just a pulling, tight, or stuck sensation. The solution to the problem is to break the individual bags free from one another as they are supposed to slide and glide on each other. For the skin on the muscles, I pull the skin in different directions making sure it moves roughly equally in all directions. If there is a direction it doesn't slide in, I give it a quick thrust in that direction to try to break it free. Other treatments that work well for this are skin rolling and slide cupping.

In particular, muscles can get stuck together post injury. I use the same principle as I do for the skin: I feel for one muscle moving past the other. If it isn't moving as much as I expect I use quick pushes or a grab it and shake it briskly to try to shake it free.

When a ligament, tendon, or muscle heals the connective tissue heals in a more disorganized manner, instead of parallel fibers, the fibers can go in more random directions. Ideally the body, on its own, remodels the structure to its initial shape, but sometimes you have to help it out. A type of massage technique called deep friction massage or cross friction massage can help. You vigorously push back and forth over the tender structure with the motion being perpendicular to the fibers.

FIBROMYALGIA

The word is derived from the Latin: "fibro" = fibrous tissues, "my" = muscles, and "algia" = pain. It is commonly described as widespread muscle and tissue pain. It was first thought that these people must have something wrong with their muscles but it was later found that the muscles and fibrous tissue seemed to be normal. The current understanding is that it is caused by the central nervous system. It is basically a case of central sensation/chronic pain syndrome, affecting multiple regions of the body at once. The brain can be so sensitive that I've heard it described as a full-body migraine. It used to be diagnosed using a map of common tender sites and a pressure/tenderness sensor called an algometer. If you were overly tender in enough of the common sites, you were diagnosed with fibromyalgia. Nowadays, the diagnosis is made with a questionnaire the patient answers.[34] If you score enough points on the questionnaire then you could be diagnosed with fibromyalgia. It is supposed to be a diagnosis of exclusion though. They are supposed to rule out all other causes of your problems before diagnosing fibromyalgia but that can be a timely and difficult endeavor.

This is a poorly understood diagnosis and its patients are often poorly managed, often just prescribed a lifetime of

---

[34] Fibromyalgia questionnaire: https://www.rcplondon.ac.uk/file/36231/download

drugs. If they develop any actual muscle pains/injuries, their new pains are disregarded as just being more fibromyalgia pain. Patients feel like their providers have given up on them. Fibromyalgia is treated like a lifetime diagnosis. Once you are diagnosed, you will always have it forever, and to the credit of the current medical system, that is the way it normally works out. But it is curable—some of my patients have resumed normal lives.

I find treating fibromyalgia as just a widespread chronic pain syndrome is more accurate and useful. While there is growing evidence that there is a genetic component predisposing some individuals to chronic pain syndromes and there are correlations to having previous emotional and physical traumas, this does not mean that having a chronic pain syndrome/fibromyalgia is a lifelong or constant issue. It might be more work for some than others to return to normal.

Like in normal chronic pain syndromes, they catastrophize (imagine the worst in terms of structural damage, or possible pain) and have fear avoidance (avoid moving or activities for fear of pain). Just touching the skin can be painful. Movements can be painful. Just like chronic pain syndromes, mental health counseling can play a major role. Any treatment that involves improving their confidence in their body and reducing fear and anxiety can be helpful. This may involve exercise, chiropractors, acupuncturists, physiotherapists, religion/God/church, mental health counselors, etc.

The reduced movement and deconditioning can also cause muscle knots which can be persistent pain generators. This pain is amplified by their condition. These muscle knots need to be worked out to eventually get them pain free. Correcting bad habits, improving muscle coordination, and re-conditioning muscles/tendons are also necessary to get them back to normal where a good personal trainer, exercise plan, physiotherapist, and/or exercise-focused chiropractor can help.

In particular, Tai Chi has been found to be one of the most helpful exercises. The lack of activities can result in poor coordination of muscles and the slow motions of Tai Chi is a great way to improve muscle coordination and improve the brains confidence in the body gradually, whereas quick movements might trigger fear that the patient might injure themselves, resulting in increased pain and muscle spasms preventing movement. Confidence is a big issue, whether it is pain lifting the arm or painful spasm when trying to bend forward. Assuming all muscle knots have already been worked out and the remaining pain is from central sensitization, it is possible, sometimes within a single session, to get these motions pain free with some patience: bending forward just 10 degrees slowly at first, then repeating at faster speeds until you have full confidence that it feels good and strong, then slowing down and increasing the distance and practicing there. Sometimes this process takes multiple days/sessions, particularly if the muscle coordination is really bad.

 This condition is related to headaches, fatigue, and depression which should be treated concurrently. There seems to be genetic and possibly a hormone connection as well. The more overweight you are, the worse it is.[35] Diet changes can help with a lot of these things and, sure enough, reduced calorie, low FODMAP, and raw vegetarian diets improved quality of life, quality of sleep, anxiety, depression, and/or inflammatory biomarkers in some people diagnosed with fibromyalgia.[36] (Note that not all diets have been tested so other diets might help you).

Vibration can have an almost magical effect on this type of pain. If I'm working on a muscle knot in someone's glutes (butt) it is common for the pain to spread to the tailbone and/or down the back of the thigh. In some individuals they have said the pain travels to their head and feet. I normally put them right away on a vibration plate or use a quickly vibrating massager and afterwards, when I continue the treatment, the pain only spreads a regular amount. It can also be useful for allodynia (pain to a non-painful stimulus), when just touching the skin or just moving the joint passively is painful when I know it shouldn't be. Overstimulating all the mechanical sensors with vibration seems to have a dampening effect on the pain, bringing it closer to normal levels, and resetting the pain threshold of the receptors.

---

[35] Núñez-Nevárez K, López-Betancourt A, Cisneros-Pérez V, et al. Relationship Between Weight and Severity of Fibromyalgia. *Mo Med.* 2023;120(1):83-88.

[36] Silva AR, Bernardo A, Costa J, et al. Dietary interventions in fibromyalgia: a systematic review. *Ann Med.* 2019;51(sup1):2-14. doi:10.1080/07853890.2018.1564360

HYPERMOBILITY

Some people have chronically stiff backs/necks and are prone to their back/necks "going out" with associated muscle spasms. Some feel their muscles are just always tight and massages are just a waste of time because their muscles tighten up right after a massage. This presentation is common in any chronic pain syndrome but, counterintuitively, hypermobile people are at an increased risk.[37]

Hypermobile individuals have extra laxity in their ligaments, allowing their joints to go further than average. There are 2 types of joint stability: structural and functional. Structural is from the shape of the bones and from the ligaments. This limits the extreme motion of the joint. Functional stability involves the coordination of the muscles that control the joint. While young and active, hypermobile patients don't experience neck pain/stiffness but through a sedentary lifestyle and/or an initial injury (sprain, whiplash, crick in neck, disc herniation, etc.), the lack of movement or lack of movement variety can decondition the tissues and reduce the robustness of the brain's control/coordination of the small muscles that control the joints. With the lack of coordination of the muscles: missing

---

[37] Scheper MC, de Vries JE, Verbunt J, Engelbert RH. Chronic pain in hypermobility syndrome and Ehlers-Danlos syndrome (hypermobility type): it is a challenge. *J Pain Res.* 2015;8:591-601. Published 2015 Aug 20. doi:10.2147/JPR.S64251

a step or turning their head sharply can cause an uncoordinated motion of the spinal segments. The body panics and locks things down with the longer/bigger neck muscles. Even after this muscle spasm subsides the body maintains a state of high alert and tries to protect the neck by keeping those muscles tight and stiff, which is counterintuitive because hypermobile people were often the most flexible in their youth.

What can they do to fix this problem?

Relaxing tight muscles via a chiropractor or massage therapist can help for the stiffness, but it won't help the lack of functional stability, so the stiffness will eventually return. Chiropractic spinal manipulations can help improve the brain's control of the spine because by manipulating the spine, tons of information about the joint is sent to the brain from mechanical sensors in the neck, helping the brain relearn about the neck. Ultimately, rehabilitation exercises with a chiropractor or a physiotherapist is the best long-term solution. Retraining the body on the coordinated use of the muscles will prevent further injuries/spasms and allow these chronic neck pain sufferers to resume a normal life again.

How to identify if you are hypermobile?

Ehlers Danlos is a hypermobility condition. It is sometimes diagnosed clinically if there are enough clinical findings but the best test for hypermobility conditions is a genetic test. The altered genes lead to stretchier collagen, the building block of skin, ligaments, and tendons. Hypermobile people are often thin and tall. They might have more stretchy and more velvety skin. They might require more local anesthetic for dental procedures or minor surgery like mole removal. They normally score 5 or more on the Beighton scale test which gives one point for each limb that can do the following: thumb to forearm, elbows or knees 10 degrees past 180 degrees, both palms touching the floor when touching their toes, and bending the pinky finger backwards past 90 degrees.

A BIT ABOUT RESEARCH IN HEALTHCARE

We love to point to a research paper and know, definitely and objectively, a truth about the world. Sadly, healthcare research sucks, particularly when it comes to anything non-drug related. Let us first talk about the best research and where most research fails.

The best research uses lots of participants. It has a very clear condition being treated and a clear demographic group who ideally don't have any other conditions that complicate matters. The demographic group could try to replicate society with all ages and genders or specific like elite, male soccer players ages 30-35. There should be clear measurements/outcome markers for both establishing the diagnosis and determining success. There should be a placebo in place for comparison. Ideally, even the clinicians and statisticians are blinded to which group is the placebo group and which is the treatment group.

No research is perfect. Even seemingly perfect studies have flaws that you have to work with. It is very often that subgroups within studies respond differently: people's livers process drugs differently, people have different lifestyles, maybe weight plays a role, some people will have other conditions not checked for which can seriously complicate matters, etc.

Let us imagine a study on a knee exercise for arthritis as diagnosed on X-ray, and we're going to rate their pain and their self-reported functional ability. How do you have a placebo? You can have a comparison treatment, or a non-treatment group but how do you have a true placebo group: a group of people who think they are getting exercises but actually aren't. You also can't blind the practitioner as to what treatment the patient is getting. Unlike drugs, there is no money to be made in finding an effective exercise, so who is funding this? Can you even pay the participants or the practitioners? You might have thousands in a drug study, but you are lucky to find exercise studies with more than 50 people in them. So maybe in a given study, there is statistically no difference with this exercise, but what about sub groups? If one third got better, one third got worse, and one third didn't change, then on average, the research study would show no result! The exercise might not be universally applicable because the study didn't keep track of who had muscle atrophy going into the study, how active each individual was, what they do for a living, etc. An overall average doesn't tell the whole story. Research, in general, doesn't take into account how different every individual's situation can be. Not only do things that physios, chiros, and acupuncturists do have poor quality research but nutraceuticals, botanicals, and supplements also have poor quality studies. An additional complication for botanical research and for the general public is you often can't trust the bottles you find on the shelf to contain what they say they contain.

Let us now talk about some potentially misleading positive research. People often get better over time with most conditions. Without taking this into account or comparing to a placebo or non-treatment group, this can make the treatment being researched seem much more effective than it is: "Wow, 100% of the people with an arm fracture no longer had one at the 2-year follow-up after taking this one special pill. This pill must have a 100% success rate at fixing broken bones!" I read a research paper recently studying the effect of custom heel-lift orthotics on back pain.[38] One hundred percent of people had no back pain when they checked on them 2 years later! Fire the spine surgeons! Close the physiotherapy businesses! Send the chiros back to school to learn how to code! We have found the solution to all back pain with a 100% success rate! Ugh… If you look at more studies you will get a better picture that orthotics have no effect or a small effect on back pain depending on the study.[39] One type of research paper is the "case study" which describes the treatment of just one patient. Normally they are written involving conditions and/or treatments that do not have thorough research on them or the patient presentation itself is more unique. When it comes to an ob-

---

[38] D'Amico M, Kinel E and Roncoletta P (2022) Leg Length Discrepancy and Nonspecific Low Back Pain: 3-D Stereophotogrammetric Quantitative Posture Evaluation Confirms Positive Effects of Customized Heel-Lift Orthotics. *Front. Bioeng. Biotechnol.* 9:743132. doi: 10.3389/fbioe.2021.743132

[39] Chuter, V., Spink, M., Searle, A. et al. The effectiveness of shoe insoles for the prevention and treatment of low back pain: a systematic review and meta-analysis of randomised controlled trials. *BMC Musculoskelet Disord* 15, 140 (2014). https://doi.org/10.1186/1471-2474-15-140

scure or new type of treatment, they are often only supporting research but... they are often only written in cases with
positive results.

No research is perfect, so what should you do, particularly,
if you aren't an expert? Look for a meta-analysis, a systematic review, or a narrative review. These types of research
papers look at all the available research studies and try to
compile/summarize the research to make it more usable. I
didn't want this book to be a textbook, so I actually limited
my use of citations, using them only when I quote a number
or to support a claim that might need more support than
just my clinical experience/specialist training. I tried to
choose representative and relatively recent systematic reviews or narrative reviews, which would encapsulate most
of the research.

Application of research is also slow. Sometimes physicians
are resistant to change. Sometimes there is no alternative,
so an archaic treatment is better than no treatment. There
is a hint of truth in almost all treatments though, so even
relatively bad treatments can still have their place. Therapeutic ultrasound became very popular and, for a time, was
found in every physiotherapist's office. The preponderance
of evidence strongly suggests it is no more effective than a
placebo, inferior to other treatments, or at best similar to a

hot pack.[40,41,42] Some physios either aren't up to date on the research, are using it instead of a hot pack, or for the placebo effect. Antidepressants, particularly SSRI's, are now well understood to have little benefit over placebo for mild and moderate depression patients (approximately 90% of depression), have a risk of adverse events, and may result in withdrawal symptoms when trying to stop.[43] But you can't prescribe a placebo, so what is the doctor supposed to do?[44] Research would suggest avoiding using cortisone unless absolutely necessary for tendon pain because even if it does give relief, it is short term only and cortisone is bad for tendon health but doctors still often use it.[45]

---

[40] Haile G, Hailemariam TT, Haile TG. Effectiveness of Ultrasound Therapy on the Management of Chronic Non-Specific Low Back Pain: A Systematic Review. *J Pain Res.* 2021;14:1251-1257. Published 2021 May 17. doi:10.2147/JPR.S277574

[41] Freiwald J, Magni A, Fanlo-Mazas P, et al. A Role for Superficial Heat Therapy in the Management of Non-Specific, Mild-to-Moderate Low Back Pain in Current Clinical Practice: A Narrative Review. *Life (Basel).* 2021;11(8):780. Published 2021 Aug 2. doi:10.3390/life11080780

[42] Aiyer R, Noori SA, Chang KV, et al. Therapeutic Ultrasound for Chronic Pain Management in Joints: A Systematic Review. *Pain Med.* 2020;21(7):1437-1448. doi:10.1093/pm/pnz102

[43] Yuan Z, Chen Z, Xue M, Zhang J, Leng L. Application of antidepressants in depression: A systematic review and meta-analysis. *J Clin Neurosci.* 2020;80:169-181. doi:10.1016/j.jocn.2020.08.013

[44] "St. John's wort" has similar effectiveness to SSRI's for depression with fewer side effects and doesn't require a prescription. See the SSRI section later in the book for more information. Exercise and counseling work well too.

[45] Coombes BK, Bisset L, Vicenzino B. Efficacy and safety of corticosteroid injections and other injections for management of tendinopathy: a systematic review of randomised controlled trials. *Lancet.* 2010;376(9754):1751-1767. doi:10.1016/S0140-6736(10)61160-9

PART 2:
LISTS

TYPES OF HEALTH PROFESSIONALS

Knowing who to get help from can be half the battle. Sadly, there are a lot of variations between practitioners, so you might have to try a few or ask a few questions to find the right one. In general, if you aren't being re-evaluated often and/or if the treatment remains the same without any improvement in your condition, it is time to start asking questions or to seek another opinion. Take ownership of your healthcare. You are the only specialist in you. You need to find someone to collaborate with. As mentioned in the book's introduction, every practitioner might view your problems through the lens of their experience and clinical training. You might have to navigate the different practitioners to resolve your problems adequately. Hence, this section will educate you on the most common health practitioners.

Chiropractors

Chiropractors are health professionals who specialize in conservative (non-pharmaceutical, non-surgical) management and treatment of nerve, muscle, and joint disorders/injuries. In particular, they specialize in traditional chiropractic adjustments (joint mobilization/manipulation) of the spine (neck and back) and other joints of the body. They may incorporate rehabilitation exercises, physical therapy modalities (like electrical stimulation), massage, acupuncture, cupping, lifestyle/dietary modifications, and/or nutritional/botanical supplements. They are trained in taking and reading radiographs (X-rays) which are often necessary in determining whether an injury is safe to treat conservatively or whether surgical intervention is necessary. They sometimes work in hospitals or multidisciplinary clinics, but they most often open their own small clinics. Chiropractors are very common in the United States and Canada with densities ranging from about 800 to 10,000 people per chiropractor depending on the city. There can be significant overlap between chiropractors and physiotherapists, naturopaths, massage therapists, acupuncturists, and osteopaths.

There is a national standard in Canada and the United States for science education, clinical experience, radiograph interpreting proficiency, ability to diagnose, and knowledge of when to refer cases when necessary. The curriculum is similar between a medical doctor and a chiropractor. Most chiropractors may have more orthopedics and neurology class-hours but less pharmacology and internal medicine class-hours compared to medical doctors. Where they went to school and what state they practice in can influence the typical chiropractor. I was trained in Oregon where chiropractors are primary care physicians, and I learned some minor surgery and obstetrics. Chiropractors at a school where they have to memorize the teachings of the earliest chiropractors may have an almost religious belief in the power of the chiropractic adjustment and may use them as their only treatment technique. Depending on the country, chiropractors may only have a bachelors or a master's degree. In some countries, the term is unregulated and anybody can call themselves a chiropractor.

There is a schism in the profession: "subluxation-based" (traditionalists or straight chiropractors) and "evidence-based" (mixers). Ultimately, the treatments may end up similar, but traditionalists often use some language and reasoning based on the writings of the first chiropractors from 100 years ago whereas evidence-based chiropractors may use language and reasoning more consistent with the medical profession. Traditionalists tend to be spine specialists and are very proficient in traditional chiropractic techniques, whereas evidence-based chiropractors are more likely to treat extremities (arms, shoulders, knees, ankles, hips, jaw, etc.) and use other soft tissue techniques aside from the traditional chiropractic adjustments. Chiropractors don't just treat serious cases such as disc herniations or whiplash. Many people go to chiropractors for mild joint stiffness, muscle tightness, muscle aches, headaches, or poor posture. Chiropractors focusing on more traditional techniques only require 2-10 minutes per patient and may see 50-100 patients a day. While most people respond well to the chiropractic adjustments, and I've seen the treatment be curative, the limitation in treatment variety, and the limited time for treatment or evaluation, often results in progress stagnation—a seemingly never-ending series of visits for mild and temporary relief, sometimes in the hope of something changing due to a cumulative effect.

Sadly, healthcare is a business and high-volume chiropractors seeing 100 people a day can make a lot of money. While these individuals still help many people, what about the people they don't help? Chiropractors are known for pushing lengthy treatment plans and "maintenance" visits. While very profitable, an ethical health professional should always be trying to put themselves out of business. While some injuries do require a lengthy recovery, most patients don't **require** continued care the for rest of their life. Some people's history of injuries and current physical demands on their body may **benefit** from continued and regular support from a chiropractor, acupuncturist, physiotherapist, personal trainer, etc. Some people love getting "cracked." **If the only thing the chiropractor is doing is cracking your back and you don't feel you are progressing, get another health professional's help** (chiropractor or otherwise). Taking time to really listen to patients and modifying the treatment plan visit-to-visit to maximize recovery isn't a financially feasible treatment model, but there are health professionals out there who choose to make less money but help people more thoroughly.

Chiropractors are more prone to using archaic, pseudo-science explanations and treatment systems (such as Applied Kinesiology) which I think discredits the field as a whole. Most pseudoscience treatments or evaluation systems have a kernel of truth to them. Chiropractors aren't the only ones who might use disproven pseudo-scientific tests: nutritionists, naturopaths, "natural healers", "magnetic healers", and massage therapists can also knowingly or unknowingly use unscientific or unfounded techniques or explanations. While the explanations may irk me, what matters is if they are helping the patient.

Chiropractors and medical doctors can be the worst for causing chronic pain syndromes. A typical strategy for chiropractors is to X-ray every patient and show them all the little things that are wrong. Similarly for medical doctors, they find one thing on X-ray and, "Aha! There is your problem." **X-ray and MRI imaging findings do not correlate very well with pain.** Lots of those imaging findings may be normal to see in pain-free individuals. But the thought of the structure being bad—the mental image of bones grinding into one another—this can lead to central sensitization and can ramp up someone's pain causing a chronic pain syndrome to develop. I think osteoarthritis should be renamed to "normal age-related bony changes" due to the poor correlation with pain and the high likelihood of finding it in pain-free joints.[46]

What is a "chiropractic subluxation"?

The "old school" thinking of chiropractic was bones-out-of-place. The medical term for a bone out of place is subluxation which refers to a partial or incomplete dislocation. The "garden hose theory" was that if a bone is out of place, it clamps down on the nerve, causing nerve-type symptoms down the path of the nerve like someone stepping on a garden hose, affecting the flow of water. Some even have a religious interpretation: that God's innate intelligence flows through the nerves, and unrestricted flow is necessary to prevent dis-ease (spelled this way on purpose to reinforce

---

[46] I want to be clear that sometimes the findings on X-ray or MRI do explain the pain. There is an increased likelihood of pain statistically if there is nasty stuff on your images but the increased likelihood may be much less than you would expect.

that the lack of flow/balance/ease is the cause of the problem rather than something structural or biological). They believe innate intelligence ensures optimum body function and all or most problems stem from a lack of nerve flow. Therefore, chiropractors can fix the flow and thereby fix almost any problem. I heard an old-school chiropractor's son was bitten by a poisonous snake near his thumb and the first thing his father did was crack his neck, corresponding to the nerves that lead to that part of the hand!

Nowadays, chiropractors focus on joints that aren't moving well, and there is a shift to call a joint that isn't moving well a "joint dysfunction" rather than a subluxation because it isn't necessarily out-of-place. Severe spinal issues can either directly compress nerves, irritate nerves chemically through inflammation, or impact the blood flow to the nerves so there may be some truth to the "garden hose theory." Most of the time, a stiff joint is just a stiff joint, and the problem at the elbow is a problem at the elbow and not a compressed nerve at the neck.

How to find a chiropractor who isn't a quack?

Chiropractors can be known for pushing for regular, frequent visits and for using fear compliance: "Unless you come back regularly, your pain will come back." Many of these chiropractors are more traditional as they focus solely on chiropractic adjustments (joint manipulations). When you limit yourself only to one tool, then they limit their ability to help people whose problems don't conform to that treatment. Because they perform it much more often, they are often the best at traditional chiropractic techniques. If your problems don't respond to a simple "crack" of the spine, then you have to be more selective of your chiropractor. The Joint is a chiropractic chain that only does chiropractic adjustments with quick 5 minutes visits.

You might look for chiropractors who advertise soft tissue work and rehab. Airrosti is a chiropractic chain that spends 1 hour per patient, focusing on soft tissue work and exercises.

Where they went to school might matter. I went to the University of Western States in Oregon. It is known as one of the most evidence-based schools. We had a journal club where we were reading research papers whereas at other schools they learned more "chiropractic philosophy" and additional traditional chiropractic techniques. Life Chiropractic College would be closer to the other end of the spectrum.

If they belong to a chiropractic organization, that can also be a hint. The International Chiropractic Association (ICA), is a traditionalist chiropractor advocacy group, whereas the American Chiropractic Association (ACA) is an advocacy group more in line with evidence-based chiropractors.

There are also chiropractic specialties where the chiropractor does at least a master's equivalent of postdoctoral studies and/or a three-year residency. I'm a board-certified chiropractic neuromusculoskeletal medicine specialist. Here the term medicine is used as "the science or practice of the diagnosis, treatment, and prevention of disease"[47] instead of as a synonym for drugs. These chiropractors specialize in diagnosis and management of nerve, muscle, and skeletal problems. These specialists used to be referred to as chiropractic orthopedists, so you may find that term still being used. A similarly trained chiropractor would use DIANM, FIANM, DACO, FACO, DABCO next to their name. A chiropractic sports physician might also be a good choice, since they will be an expert in exercise training and rehabilitation. They use CCSP or DACBSP next to their name. Chiropractic rehab specialists use DACRB. There are great chiropractors without a specialty too, and having extra education doesn't mean they will be great, but it might be a good place to start.

Doctors of Traditional Chinese Medicine (Acupuncturists)

Traditional Chinese Medicine (TCM) practitioners might use a variety of treatment techniques: moxibustion (burning a special herb), TDP Lamp (infrared heating), cupping, tui na (massage), gua sha (massage with an edged jade/plastic/wood tool), herbal remedies, and acupuncture.

The most unique part of TCM is the diagnosis system which focuses on organs, elements, yin/yang energy, and blood. The organs in TCM have different roles from modern medi-

---

[47] Merriam-Webster. (n.d.). Medicine. In Merriam-Webster.com dictionary. Retrieved July 4, 2023, from https://www.merriam-webster.com/dictionary/medicine

cine. The practitioner knows that the TCM organ and the actual organ aren't necessarily the same thing. The TCM organ represents a set of functions of the body. The patient's symptoms go into creating a TCM diagnosis which might not make sense to an MD, but is required to create a TCM treatment plan based on this diagnosis. The intermediate step of the diagnosis doesn't need to make sense to western medicine as long as the treatment helps the patient with their symptoms. As an example, the spleen in western medicine controls the level of white blood cells, red blood cells, and platelets. In TCM, it is responsible for transformation and transportation. It transforms food into nutritive essence which is sent to the heart and lungs to be transformed into blood, and qi and is connected to a balanced earth element.

The diagnosis aims to address the whole body's problems, not only muscle stiffness or pain. The practitioner will take a detailed health history and ask about your issues such as sleep, digestion, temperature sensitivities, etc. They will look at your tongue and feel your pulse.

Acupuncture has some evidence to support its use for musculoskeletal pain relief and is sometimes even covered by medical insurance.[48] Placing needles into tight muscles or even nasty muscle knots is an effective way at relaxing muscles and reducing the size of the muscle knots. It can be so comfortable that people can fall asleep full of needles. The needle might pinch going in but either feels like nothing or there is a sense of pressure.

---

[48] See the treatment section of this book for more information.

Physiotherapists

There can be a lot of overlap between an evidence-based chiropractor and a physiotherapist. In the US, physiotherapists also obtain a doctorate. They learn the same neurological and orthopedic exams and more rehab protocols compared with the average chiropractor. Whereas exercises may be an afterthought in most chiropractic programs and chiropractors might have to obtain post-doctoral training, physiotherapists come equipped with an excellent repertoire of rehabilitation exercises right out of school. They are normally better equipped for sports injuries as well. They can learn grade 5 joint mobilizations (chiropractic adjustments) too. A chiropractor might start with adjustments whereas a physio might start with a grade 3 or 4 joint mobilization or a stretch instead. Some chiropractors don't spend any time on rehab, but a physio is almost guaranteed to spend time on rehab. Physiotherapists do have a special niche for post-surgical rehab, which most chiropractors have no experience with. Physiotherapists work in hospitals and private clinics compared to chiropractors who are rarely found in a hospital setting. Physiotherapists are also less likely to learn pseudoscience quackery compared to a chiropractor.

Just like there can be quite the variety in chiropractors, there can be a variety in physiotherapists as well. Sadly, you might have to try a few to find one with the right strategy for your problem. How many times have I heard a patient say they've tried physiotherapy and it didn't work, only to hear that they only received a hot pack and electrical stimulation. I've heard of other physiotherapists that never re-evaluate the patient and just do the same exercises again and again despite not seeing any more improvement. The best physios tend to use a variety of strategies which they modify visit to visit based on the patient's progress and response.

Personal Trainers

There are no license requirements for personal trainers unlike for chiropractors, physiotherapists, medical doctors, etc. In theory, anyone can claim to be a personal trainer. Most gyms hire someone with some sort of certification through a program accredited by the National Commission for Certifying Agencies (NCCA) which requires an exam and continuing education requirements. Many of these individuals do have bachelor degrees in kinesiology, exercise science, biology, etc. (What else are you going to do with such a degree?) The certified personal trainer credentials have the organization's name attached to them like "ISSA-CPT." Some of these programs can be completed in a month and may be only 20 hours of study. They often add on some health coach/nutrition training as well. For a pain-free individual, I see no problems with personal trainers, but for the most part, they aren't trained in rehabilitation or how to deal with pain. They likely don't know how to recondition a weakened tendon. They can sometimes miss some subtleties in exercises as well. For example, they might do hip abductor exercises or quad exercises, but the individual might have a muscle imbalance where one hip abductor is weak/deactivated or one out of the four quad muscles is weaker. They often don't tailor the exercises to that level of detail whereas a physiotherapist or an exercise-minded chiropractor might.

Massage therapists

Depending on the state/province/country you are in, massage therapists might be licensed or not. Sometimes these licenses are easy to obtain, and sometimes require years of training. It is very often that people go to a massage therapist for muscle pains, headaches, etc. They are not trained to evaluate what is causing your pain, nor necessarily how to adapt the message to target your pain. They can target any muscle you point to but they will likely use their trained massage techniques instead of something more clinical: "Oh, you feel tight there? Let me do extra Swedish massage there." An achy tight muscle responds well to massage but muscle knots do not. They respond to compression. Some muscles are best worked on while moving that part of the body like the quadratus lumborum or pectoralis minor, but the massage often misses those muscles, not for lack of trying on the part of the massage therapist, but because they require body movement to treat all their fibers and for the duration of a traditional massage you are just lying there. In particular, for chronic muscle tightness, if you find your neck or back stiffens up within 1-12 hours, then chances are you need rehab of the neck and/or back more than stretches/massages. If the brain is worried about you hurting the neck/back then it wants to keep the muscles tight.

Psychologists/Psychiatrists/Counselors

Someone once told me that a psychologist is a friend you pay for. These are people who you will open up to, will have deep conversations with, and will offer advice. There are multiple types of strategies for tackling the same mental problem, and people have different personalities. Don't stay with a health counselor you don't jive with or one that you feel isn't helping you. This is a chronic pain book, and anyone with chronic pain should consider whether counseling is right for them. The academic literature is all over the place as every study uses different measurements and different treatment protocols, but the overarching consensus is that it helps, at least a subset of people, with reducing anxiety and pain while increasing functional capacity.[49,50] Cognitive behavioral therapy (CBT) has the most research done on it. Personally, I've had patients finally get pain-free after years of suffering with the help of hypnotherapy, CBT, and biofeedback therapy. The combination of physical therapy with mental health counseling can be required for the most stubborn cases of central sensitization: one treatment to get rid of muscle aches and make the body stronger and more capable, and the other treatment to work on the anxiety, worry, and fear.

---

[49] Başak, İ. N. C. E.. Systematic Review of the Comparative Effectiveness of Cognitive-Behavioural Therapies for Chronic Pain. *Journal of Cognitive-Behavioral Psychotherapy and Research*, 2020:9(3); 248-248.

[50] Chao YS, Ford C. Cognitive Behavioural Therapy for Chronic Non-Cancer Pain: A Review of Clinical Effectiveness [Internet]. *Ottawa (ON): Canadian Agency for Drugs and Technologies in Health;* 2019 Sep 16. Available from: https://www.ncbi.nlm.nih.gov/books/NBK549547/

Medical Doctors

The typical doctor. Basic medical education followed by a residency where the doctor learns their specialty. Heavy in pharmacology but, in general, lighter in musculoskeletal issues than the other health professionals. Often trained to see things in terms of surgery, injections, or pills. In general, the average clinic doctor has a poor ability to differentiate muscle pain from nerve pain, tendon pain from osteoarthritis pain, etc. Specialists can be much better, but remember that they are looking at your problem through the lens of their specialty. The neurologist is sure there is a nerve issue… but is that all you have? Does it explain all your symptoms? They might not be thinking that far. The surgeon is looking for a reason/justification to do surgery. This isn't necessarily malicious of the practitioner. When you go for a consultation with a surgeon, the question they hear is, "Could surgery maybe help?"

While widely seen as more trustworthy and science-based compared to naturopaths and chiropractors, allopathic (medical) doctors can be prone to unscientific/unfounded treatments/protocols due to: lack of research, archaic traditions/training, not being up-to-date with the latest research, or when non-pharmaceutical treatment options are best. They might prescribe a drug or give an injection that, with more recent research, has been proven to work poorly or is inferior to a non-pharmaceutical option. A pet peeve of mine in obstetrics: inducing labor with Pitocin or stirrup use for delivery aren't better for the patient![51,52]

Osteopaths

Osteopaths are similar to chiropractors in many ways. Both started about 100 years ago and both struggled to find a marketing niche and both were struggling not to get arrested for practicing medicine without a license. Traditional chiropractors followed nerves and were obsessed with spinal joints. Osteopaths were obsessed with the "law of the artery:" blood flow and organs. The traditional treatments often have a pulsing rhythm to them.

Doctors of Osteopathic Medicine (DOs) in all 50 states can prescribe medicine and perform surgeries. They are basically interchangeable with MDs except they have some traditional manipulative treatment techniques. They are often taught joint manipulations just like chiropractors too. Most DOs don't end up using their traditional techniques after graduation and are truly indistinguishable from MDs in how they practice. Osteopaths outside of the US cannot prescribe or perform surgery and are limited to their traditional techniques. Their training may be somewhere between that of a chiropractor and a massage therapist. Depending on the country, the term might be unregulated and they may have no formal training of licensure.

---

[51] https://evidencebasedbirth.com/evidence-birthing-positions/

[52] Espada-Trespalacios X, Ojeda F, Perez-Botella M, et al. Oxytocin Administration in Low-Risk Women, a Retrospective Analysis of Birth and Neonatal Outcomes. *Int J Environ Res Public Health.* 2021;18(8):4375. Published 2021 Apr 20. doi:10.3390/ijerph18084375

Podiatrists/Chiropodists

This is a medical specialty focusing on the feet. In the states, they will possess a doctorate in podiatric medicine. They may have undergone the training to also perform surgeries. They can help with skin and biomechanical problems. They often provide/sell custom orthotics.

Pain Management Specialists

There have been attempts to make this an official specialty in the states, but as of now, the term in the states is not protected and is used to self-describe multiple professions and multiple skill sets. It might be an orthopedic surgeon skilled in nerve ablation (killing nerves), a medical doctor knowledgeable in pain killers, a psychologist/counselor who uses cognitive behavioral therapy, or a sports medicine/orthopedic doctor skilled in injections. There are educational programs and master's degrees in pain management which often focus on the psychological aspect as well as the injection, medicine, and/or surgical interventions. Someone self-titling themselves as a pain management specialist doesn't hold a lot of weight to me as to whether they are truly good at trying to resolve chronic pain. They could just be giving out pills like candy. They could just be injecting everyone with cortisone, maybe without using ultrasound guidance. Having a master's degree holds more weight to me, but it is just a piece of paper, and a good family doctor taking the time to self-educate themselves and taking the time to listen to their patients could be better. A common theme in this section on health professionals is each practitioner can be different and you have to be self-informed to a certain extent and/or seek out multiple opinions. (note: There are some countries that do have pain management as an official specialty, but you still don't know what you are getting in each country as eligible professions and training varies from country to country.[53,54])

Naturopaths

Like chiropractors and osteopaths, naturopathic doctors have similar training to medical doctors. They may be recognized as primary care practitioners, and they may be able to prescribe drugs, perform injections, and perform surgeries but their scope of practice can vary state to state. In Oregon, they are primary care physicians and may act as an obstetrician or a family doctor. They can prescribe, inject, deliver babies, and perform minor surgery. The core of the profession is using natural healing. They tend to use nutrition and natural remedies before resorting to anything else. They tend to order lots of tests to determine if there are any organ issues and/or nutritional deficiencies. They are sometimes criticized for ordering too many tests and assuming everyone's problem is nutrient related and/or could be fixed by nutritional intervention (just how a surgeon tries to find explanations for someone's problems that can be helped by surgery). Research for nutraceuticals/botanical remedies are often limited in quality, if it exists at all.

---

[53] Hochberg U, Sharon H, Bahir I, Brill S. Pain Management - A Decade's Perspective of a New Subspecialty. *J Pain Res.* 2021;14:923-930. Published 2021 Apr 9. doi:10.2147/JPR.S303815

[54] Status of Pain Management and Credentialing

Sometimes the profession is criticized for not being evidence-based enough.

Functional Medicine Practitioners

This is a type of medicine popularized by Dr. Mark Hyman. A superficial understanding of the field would suggest that the practitioners just push for plant based, whole-food diets, but it is more involved than that. This emerging field is... basically what naturopaths have been doing for decades. They often order lots of tests: blood, fecal, saliva, genetic tests, etc. They are looking for trace element, vitamin, and mineral deficiencies; looking for food sensitivities; and promoting non-pharmaceutical remedies. The Wikipedia article says that this is an unproven pseudo-science, but there is a basis in science for everything that they do... but the research is lacking. I understand the criticism, as just because it works in a petri-dish or theoretically doesn't mean it applies in practice.

Some of their tests and prescribed solutions are often based on a chemical mechanism or on an in-vitro study (petri dish), but ideally there would be sufficiently robust human studies because our body has so many interacting systems. So, even if there is some scientific reasoning, there is sometimes no evidence that that holds true for a patient. Some functional medicine training may be done by any health professional, but some programs are reserved for doctoral level practitioners. There are educational programs popping up all over the place with master's degrees focusing on this emerging field. Most functional medicine practitioners

in the states are naturopaths, medical doctors, and chiropractors.

Lifestyle Medicine Practitioners

These physicians/professionals will likely push for lifestyle changes before jumping to medications and surgeries whenever possible. Many chronic health conditions are preventable, treatable, and/or reversible with improved diet, regular activity/exercise, restorative sleep, stress management, minimizing negative substances (tobacco, alcohol, etc.) and/or positive social connections. For example, early type-II diabetes is reversible with diet changes, but how many people out there are not told this and instead just prescribed more and more drugs?

Lifestyle medicine practitioners are most often medical physicians but could be any type of health professional, although it is particularly relevant to MDs as they receive little training in managing chronic conditions in ways that don't require surgery or drugs. This certification with the lifestyle medicine board only requires 40 hours of study plus an exam, but most of these individuals already have a doctoral level health education behind them. The training also involves some coaching techniques to help patients succeed. They will recommend plant-based diets as those diets have the best health outcomes in the research.

In the states, look for practitioners with a DipACLM, DipA-BLM, or FACLM after their name. The letters used might change in other countries as there are all sorts of international lifestyle medicine boards which share the same educational standards (I have DipIBLM).

Health and Wellness Coaches

This term is not protected so anyone can call themselves a health and/or wellness coach, but there is a certification with the National Board for Health & Wellness Coaching and this certification is recognized by the National Board of Medical Examiners. Their certification is NBHWC. The personal trainer certification organizations like ACE, ISSA, NASM, etc. have their own certifications. The scope of topics tends to match that of a lifestyle medicine practitioner: sleep, diet, avoiding negative substances, regular exercise, stress management, and positive social connections.

Nutritionists/Dieticians

The terms nutritionist and dietician are sometimes used interchangeably for someone who aids with diet advice and helps with nutritional deficiencies. Anyone can say they are a nutritionist because it is not a protected term that requires a license to practice. Some may have a 10-20-hour course, a 100-hour course, or a master's degree. Don't discount other health professionals such as chiropractors, medical doctors, naturopaths, etc., which may have similar or better training than someone with a 20-hour course. For basic nutrition advice, a 20-hour course might be sufficient. Dietician is a protected term with licensing and educational requirements. In general, a dietician is more trustworthy in

                                        BRANDON RAMAKKO

helping you tailor your diet for the treatment of a particular disease.

Magnetic (Auric) Healers

Hogwash. This type of healing influences the energy/aura by the practitioner moving their hands above a patient's body. Obviously, this doesn't have physical effects on the patient beyond a psychosomatic (mind affecting the body) placebo effect. Over a 100 years ago, they had a good track record and were a good choice compared to often lethal surgeries and possibly toxic medicinal tonics because, at the very least, they caused no harm in non-emergency situations. Nowadays, I would not visit one, but if a friend is having a beneficial effect, maybe you shouldn't burst their bubble. Interestingly, the first chiropractor was a magnetic healer before "inventing" chiropractic.

TYPES OF TREATMENTS

Homeopathy

Although the term "homeopathic remedies" is sometimes used interchangeably with natural/botanical remedies, they are not the same. Natural remedies have an active medicinal ingredient. Homeopathic concoctions/medications almost always contain no active ingredients. This is the drug equivalent of Magnetic(aura) healing. If there are no active ingredients, they are obviously safe, but any benefit relies on the placebo effect.

The original concept was "like cures like," so they would use a rash causing chemical to cure a rash. They wouldn't use the chemical directly; they would dilute it... multiple times. They incorrectly hypothesized that the more times it is diluted the stronger the effect would be. They would put one drop into a 100mL of water, then would take one drop of that and place it in 100mL of water, and they would repeat the process until they hit the desired "strength." The strength is given by how many times they have repeated the procedure. So 20c means they diluted it 20 times. At 12c or higher there likely isn't even a single molecule of the original substance (1 part in 1,000,000,000,000,000,000,000,000).

Applied Kinesiology

One of the worst examples of a treatment a chiropractor might do that discredits the entire profession is called "Applied Kinesiology" (AK). It sounds so scientific but has no relationship to the scientific field of kinesiology (the study of movement). The concept behind this evaluation method centers on using muscle strength tests to determine structural problems, internal problems, chemical problems (like food sensitivities), or mental problems. For structural problems, it can work (testing pelvis muscle strength can be a good indicator as to whether there is a problem in the pelvis) and muscle strength testing is standard in neurological and orthopedic exams.[55] The other aspects of AK have no foundation in science. Imagine holding different foods in your hand and, with each one, your muscles are tested. When you test the weakest, you conclude you are sensitive/intolerant of that food and you should avoid it. In explaining this bullshit to someone, I told them to hold out their arm. I pushed down on it firmly, then I put a piece of candy in her hand and pushed on her arm again. This time it was weaker and I told her this means you need to stay away from sugar. Even in the context of explaining it was bullshit, she said, "Are you sure it doesn't work?" It can be

---

[55] Estrázulas JA, Bueno LS, Lombardi LRO, Estrázulas JA, Fernandes TG, Baltar JA. Accuracy of the Applied Kinesiology Muscle Strength Test for Sacroiliac Dysfunction. *Rev Bras Ortop* (Sao Paulo). 2020;55(3):293-297. doi:10.1055/s-0039-1700832

convincing, and chances are, she should avoid sugar anyways. When double-blinded studies are done, this evaluation is no better than random chance for diagnosis.[56]

Red Light Therapy

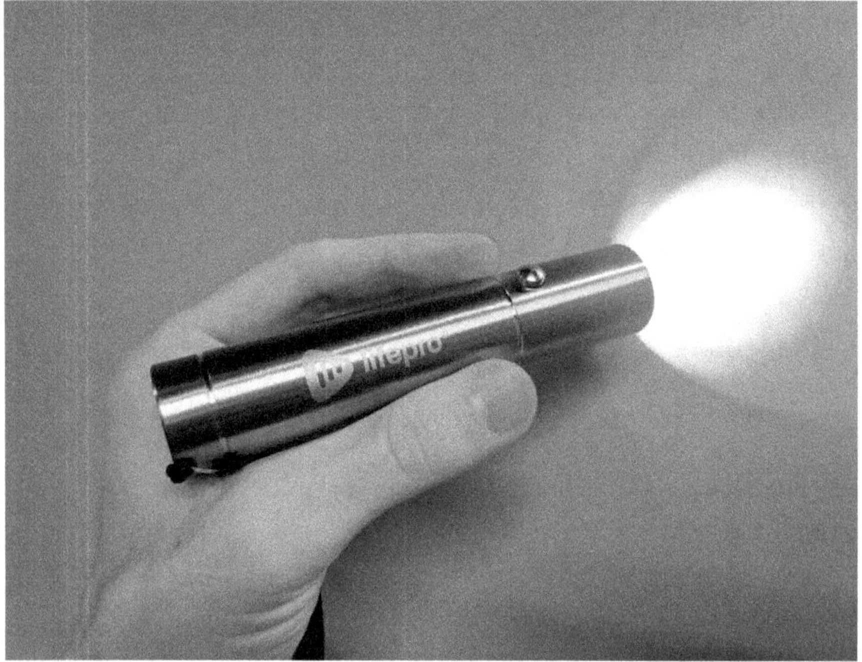

This uses very bright red lights to help with healing/pain.
This used to be called cold laser therapy because they used
lasers instead of LED lights and "cold" was referring to the
fact the dose of light is not enough to heat the skin. This
therapy is different from a heat lamp. Since the switch from
lasers to LEDs and the mass production for the consumer

[56] Schwartz SA, Utts J, Spottiswoode SJ, et al. A double-blind, randomized
study to assess the validity of applied kinesiology (AK) as a diagnostic tool
and as a nonlocal proximity effect. *Explore* (NY). 2014;10(2):99-108.
doi:10.1016/j.explore.2013.12.002

  BRANDON RAMAKKO

market, the price has dropped drastically. Whereas you used to have to buy them from medical supply stores, they can be found in pharmacies, box stores, and Amazon. We have 2 machines in our clinic and the older one was $5,000 USD and the newer one was $90 USD. Obviously, the people selling the lights will say it fixes everything, and it is a very safe treatment, as long as you don't shine it in your eyes too much.

Although the research is of fairly low quality in general, it has relatively strong evidence for help with inflammation from an acute injury (ankle sprain, tendon tear, etc.).[57] If an injured patient has a joint which is hot and feels swollen, I'm likely going to be using the light on them. For more chronic issues, the quality of the evidence is also low, but some studies have found a small effect.[58] I will use the light on a tendinosis, but I'm typically multitasking as I'm doing it.

 Since the price has come down so far, it is a reasonable purchase to add to a family's first aid kit. It doesn't hurt to try it to treat a tendinosis or chronic joint pain.[59]

---

[57] Stergioulas A, Low-Level Laser Treatment Can Reduce Edema in Second Degree Ankle Sprains. *Journal of Clinical Laser Medicine & Surgery.* Apr 2004. 125-128. http://doi.org/10.1089/104454704774076181

[58] Tripodi, N., Feehan, J., Husaric, M. et al. The effect of low-level red and near-infrared photobiomodulation on pain and function in tendinopathy: a systematic review and meta-analysis of randomized control trials. *BMC Sports Sci Med Rehabil* 13, 91 (2021). https://doi.org/10.1186/s13102-021-00306-z

[59] Jan M Bjordal, Christian Couppé, Roberta T Chow, Jan Tunér, Elisabeth Anne Ljunggren, A systematic review of low level laser therapy with location-specific doses for pain from chronic joint disorders, *Australian Journal*

Therapeutic Ultrasound

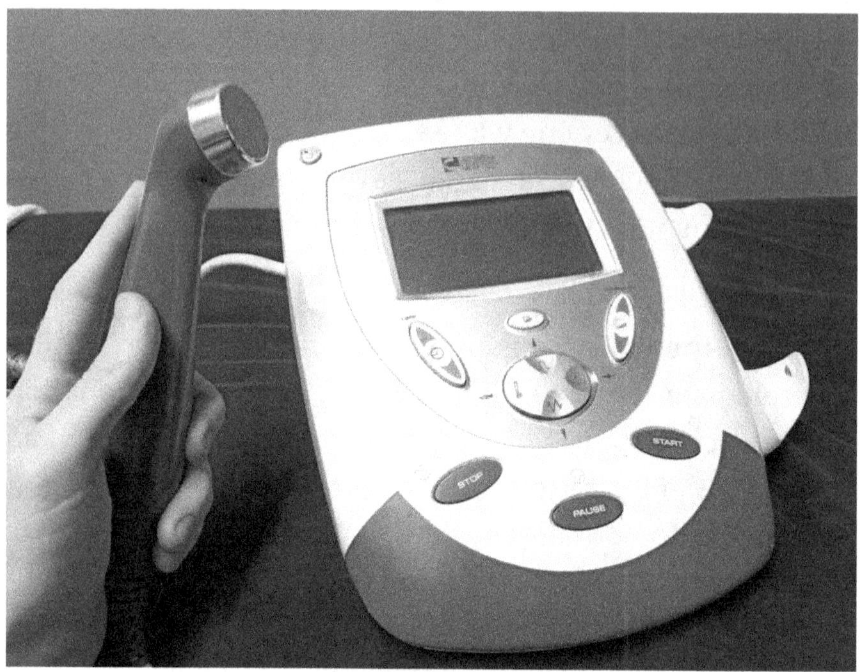

It is difficult to find a chiropractic clinic or a physiotherapist's office which doesn't have a therapeutic ultrasound machine. Ultrasound is high frequency sound above the hearing range of a human. These machines pump the sound through the tissue, shaking the cells and heating the tissue. Despite how common they are, after decades of use we now have collected a sizable amount of data on their effectiveness and the machines in these clinics are not as effective as we thought. In study after study, it has failed to be more ef-

of Physiotherapy, Volume 49, Issue 2, 2003, Pages 107-116, ISSN 0004-9514, https://doi.org/10.1016/S0004-9514(14)60127-6

fective than placebo or, in cases where it is better than placebo, there are much better alternatives.[60,61] It does provide a pleasant, deep heating sensation, and some physiotherapists still use it for a placebo and/or muscle relaxing effect (similar to using a hot pack). There is a risk if the practitioner is inattentive and delivers too much heat as they can burn the tissue lining the bones (periosteum). For some very specific conditions, it is effective, like for calcific tendinitis.[62,63]

---

[60] Robertson VJ, Baker KG. A review of therapeutic ultrasound: effectiveness studies. *Phys Ther.* 2001;81(7):1339-1350.

[61] Aiyer R, Noori SA, Chang KV, et al. Therapeutic Ultrasound for Chronic Pain Management in Joints: A Systematic Review. *Pain Med.* 2020;21(7):1437-1448. doi:10.1093/pm/pnz102

[62] Shomoto K, Takatori K, Morishita S, et al. Effects of ultrasound therapy on calcificated tendinitis of the shoulder. *J Jpn Phys Ther Assoc.* 2002;5(1):7-11. doi:10.1298/jjpta.5.7

[63] Čota S, Delimar V, Žagar I, et al. Efficacy of therapeutic ultrasound in the treatment of chronic calcific shoulder tendinitis: a randomized trial. *Eur J Phys Rehabil Med.* 2023;59(1):75-84. doi:10.23736/S1973-9087.22.07715-2

Extracorporeal Shockwave Therapy

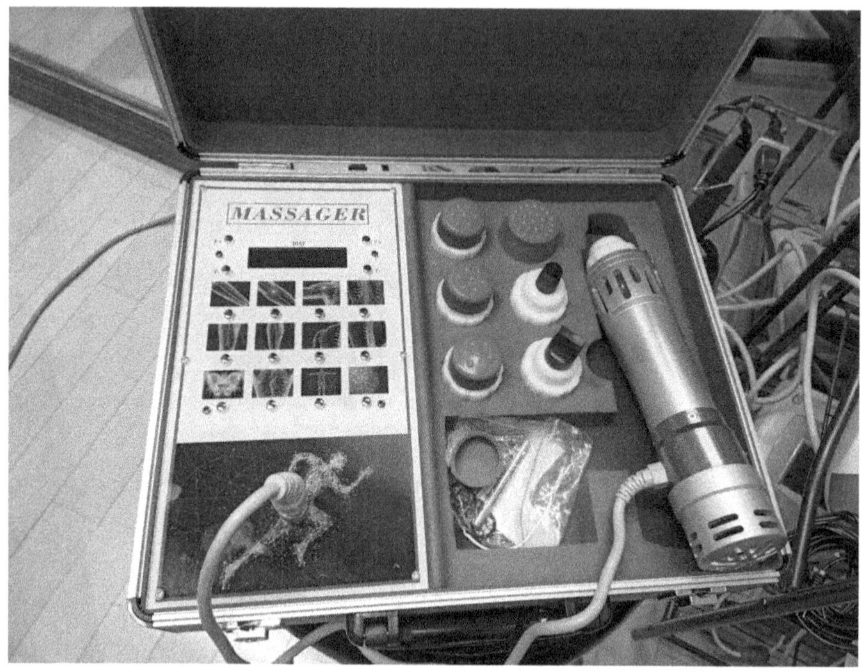

Everyone first bought therapeutic ultrasounds, then everyone bought cold lasers, and now the cool machine to get is an Extracorporeal Shockwave Therapy (EWST) machine. Initial research seems to be promising but some supposed benefits will require more research to verify. The machine vibrates the tissue somewhere between a therapeutic ultrasound machine and a percussion muscle massager. The machine accelerates a small metal "bullet" using electromagnetism or air pressure that then strikes a metal plate in contact with the patient's body. This causes a shockwave to travel into the patient's tissues. This shockwave seems to stimulate healing and building of new and/or stronger tissues. This treatment has been well established to help with bone healing, and there are signs it can help with soft tissue issues as well.[64] Tenocytes are cells within tendons responsible for making the collagen that gives the tendon its strength. They react to strong forces on the tendon, so you can imagine if a powerful shockwave goes by, that can wake up the tenocytes: "Hmmm, the body is exerting a lot of force on the tendon, I better wake up and make the tendon stronger." There is some early evidence it helps with tendon healing/strengthening/reconditioning, so it likely helps with calcific tendinitis, tendinosis, and plantar fasciosis/fasciitis.[65,66] It may be dose dependent, though, so a weaker/shorter dose might not be as effective, and it may be best paired with other treatments.[67] There is one study that found it was also effective at treating nasty muscle knots (but not more effective than ischemic compression).[68]

---

[64] Sansone V, Ravier D, Pascale V, Applefield R, Del Fabbro M, Martinelli N. Extracorporeal Shockwave Therapy in the Treatment of Nonunion in Long Bones: A Systematic Review and Meta-Analysis. *J Clin Med.* 2022;11(7):1977. Published 2022 Apr 1. doi:10.3390/jcm11071977

[65] Korakakis V, Whiteley R, Tzavara A, et al. The effectiveness of extracorporeal shockwave therapy in common lower limb conditions: a systematic review including quantification of patient-rated pain reduction. *British Journal of Sports Medicine* 2018;52:387-407.

[66] Feeney KM. The Effectiveness of Extracorporeal Shockwave Therapy for Midportion Achilles Tendinopathy: A Systematic Review. *Cureus.* 2022;14(7):e26960. Published 2022 Jul 18. doi:10.7759/cureus.26960

[67] Speed C. A systematic review of shockwave therapies in soft tissue conditions: focusing on the evidence. *Br J Sports Med.* 2014;48(21):1538-1542. doi:10.1136/bjsports-2012-091961

[68] Lee CH, Lee SU. Usefulness of Extracorporeal Shockwave Therapy on Myofascial Pain Syndrome. *Ann Rehabil Med.* 2021;45(4):261-263. doi:10.5535/arm.21128

Electrical Stimulation

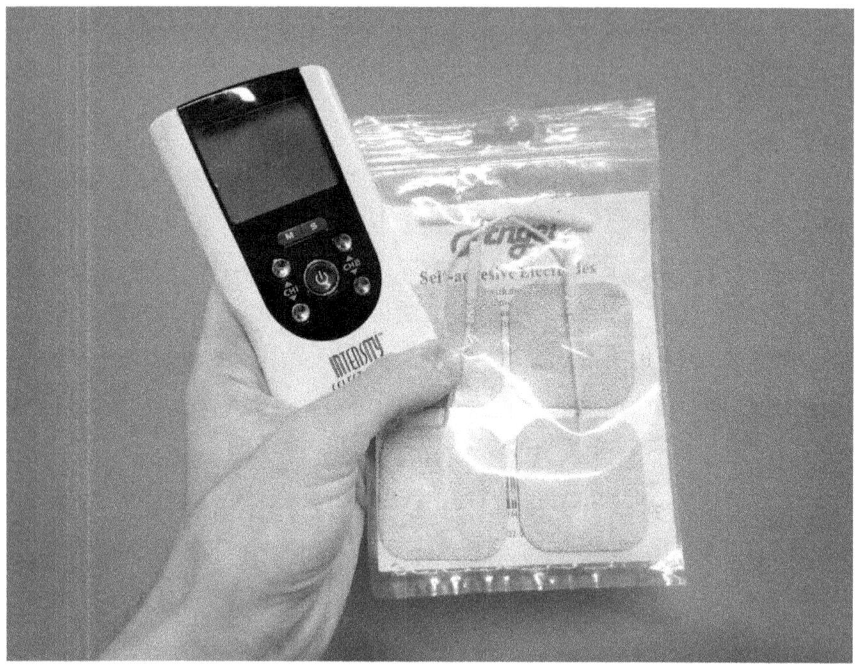

There are lots of types of electrical stimulation and even within the same type there are different settings and machines. You might run into TENS, interferential current, microcurrent, and Russian/muscle stim. For acute or chronic pain, TENS and interferential current are the most relevant, and Russian stim may aid in cases of nerve damage.

TENS numbs the nerves effectively reducing pain without drugs.[69] This effect is temporary but the reduction in pain might make it possible to do rehab exercises, or it can help

---

[69] Johnson MI, Paley CA, Jones G, Mulvey MR, Wittkopf PG. Efficacy and safety of transcutaneous electrical nerve stimulation (TENS) for acute and chronic pain in adults: a systematic review and meta-analysis of 381 studies (the meta-TENS study). *BMJ Open*. 2022;12(2):e051073. Published 2022 Feb 10. doi:10.1136/bmjopen-2021-051073

reduce anxiety/improve comfort helping to combat central sensitization. The purpose is not normally to cause muscle spasms/jumping, although, that might be an unintended consequence, particularly with TENS. TENS uses two pads and uses a frequency of about 60Hz to numb the nerves between the two pads which are normally only 2-3 inches apart. The setting is normally turned up as high as comfortable. TENS machines are cheap and can be found almost anywhere for $20-$30USD.

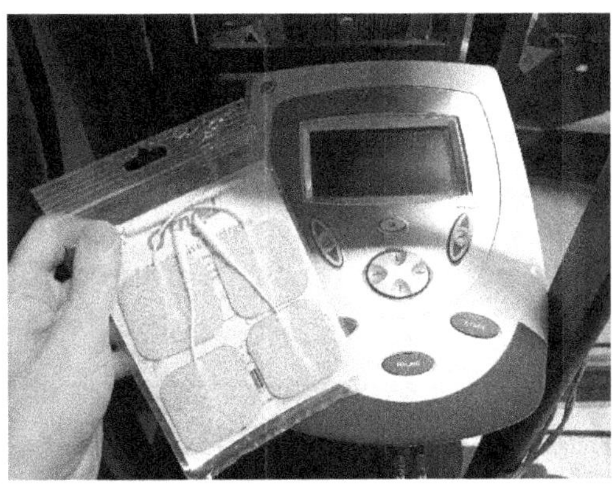

Interferential Current is a better version of TENS because it does what TENS does but in a more comfortable way.[70] I personally found it more effective and would never use TENS if interferential current was an option. The machines are more expensive and more difficult to find, normally only available from medical supply businesses to doctors and patients with prescriptions. This is the typical pain-relieving treatment at a physiotherapist or chiropractor's office.

[70] Hussein HM, Alshammari RS, Al-Barak SS, Alshammari ND, Alajlan SN, Althomali OW. A Systematic Review and Meta-analysis Investigating the Pain-Relieving Effect of Interferential Current on Musculoskeletal Pain. *Am J Phys Med Rehabil.* 2022;101(7):624-633. doi:10.1097/PHM.0000000000001870

Higher frequencies travel through the skin better than low frequencies, so with interferential current, it uses higher frequencies of around 4000Hz. This treatment requires a 4-pad set-up, making an X over the painful location. Each pair of pads has a slightly different frequency. Where the frequencies interact, they "interfere" with each other, resulting in a frequency equal to the difference between the two. So, since the 4000Hz travels more comfortably in the body, it can be turned up higher than TENS to deliver a more effective treatment at the painful site.

Russian/muscle stim uses electricity to cause muscle contractions/spasms. In particular, this is useful in someone with significant nerve compression/damage or brain damage. With nerve compression, the ability to activate the muscle is reduced. In the short term, I use Russian stim to keep the muscle from wasting away entirely. It can help with retraining as well as the patient can try to move the muscle at the same time as the electricity activates helping to retrain the brain to use the muscle to improve strength and performance.[71]

Muscle Energy Techniques

Muscle energy techniques are a class of techniques/stretches that involve activating your muscles to help your muscles relax and to improve your range of motion. I first encountered them before learning any

---

[71] Wang TJ, Sung K, Wilburn M, Allbright J. Russian Stimulation/Functional Electrical Stimulation in the Treatment of Foot Drop Resulting from Lumbar Radiculopathy: A Case Series. *Innov Clin Neurosci.* 2019;16(5-6):46-49.

　　BRANDON RAMAKKO

healthcare during gymnastics training. I'll briefly cover 3 versions: PIR, RI, and CRAC. All three strategies can be used on any muscle and can be combined with virtually any passive stretch you already like.

Post-isometric relaxation (PIR) involves stretching a muscle close to end range, to the point where you first start to feel some resistance. Then you activate the muscle you are trying to stretch for about 6 seconds. Some people debate about how much you should activate it. Some say 20% if your goal is to relax a muscle spasm and some say about 80% if you are focusing on maximizing flexibility. Regardless, after the 6 seconds, take a break for a few seconds. Maybe take a deep breath, then you'll find that you can stretch the muscle a bit further until you encounter some resistance again. The process can be repeated until there is no longer any improvement or you feel the muscle has relaxed sufficiently. For a more concrete example, let me choose a pec stretch in a doorway. I grab the edge of the doorframe and lean forward stretching my pecs. I don't go until it is painful, I just go to where I can feel the muscle is tight. Then I activate the pec muscle by trying to pull my arm forward for 6 seconds, not so much that I actually move my body. I then take a breath, then move further until the muscle starts to feel taut again and repeat the process.

Reciprocal Inhibition (RI) tricks your body into relaxing the opposite muscles to the ones you activate. If I lazily look towards my left, I go about 60 degrees until I feel a tightness at the front-right side of my neck. If I now imagine that there is something super important behind me, I need to see (I can even lead with my eyes) and I hold it for 6 seconds. Afterwards, if I lazily turn left, I can turn to about 80 degrees before feeling the tightness. When we turned left with a sense of urgency/effort, the brain then decided to relax all the muscles that turn right to make it easier for us. We can abuse this to relax any set of muscles in the body. In the posture section of the book, I mention an exercise of pulling the shoulder blades back and down 3 times for 6 seconds each with maximum safe effort. So, this exercise works to relax the opposite muscles. The opposite of back and down is up and forward so this exercise relaxes the muscles on top of the shoulder (upper traps and levator scapulae) and the muscles in the front of the shoulder (pec major and minor). RI can also be done very similarly to PIR. Using the neck rotation example, I could turn left until I first hit resistance and then block the head with my hand and push to turn left into my hand without going anywhere for 6 seconds. Afterwards, if things worked, the muscle should be relaxed. If I need more mobility, I could go further in rotation to the new location of tension and repeat. This braced version is more useful if moving your neck in extreme positions is painful, but you still want to relax some muscles. If the goal is building maximal flexibility/range-of-motion, then as a final round, you might want to push in the direction of motion to maximize the range of motion as you are activating the muscles.

Contract-Relax-Antagonist Contract (CRAC) is a combination of PIR and RI. You basically do a round (or multiple rounds) of PIR and then follow it by doing a round (or multiple rounds) of RI. This is how we were trying to achieve our splits when I did acrobatics. We called it "procedure de diable" which translates to "devil's procedure" because we were pretty aggressive with it. You don't need to be so aggressive, though, to gain some benefits.

Hot/cold

Hot and cold and two very accessible means of relief. Although, the relief can be temporary.

Heat can help muscles relax and possibly offer some pain relief. If the brain doesn't want the muscles to relax, then the muscles might tighten again. If you have muscle knots, it might take the tension off the knots, reducing pain, but it might not have any effect on eliminating the knots. Working at a comfortable temperature can help prevent shoulder muscle knots as you won't be shivering and hunched, trying to stay warm. Heat increases blood flow to an area. If an area is swollen/inflamed, you don't want more fluid there, so heat is to be avoided.

Cold was the go-to for injuries, then went out of favor, and now it is okay again. This book is about chronic pain and not about acute injuries, but when you hurt something seriously, they used to use the acronym RICE for: Rest, Ice, Compress, and Elevate. Now they use POLICE for Protect, Optimally Load, Ice, Compress, Elevate. "Rest" was removed because too much rest requires more rehab later. The Ice, Compress, and Elevate is for swelling control. Cold/ice drives fluid away from the area. Cold/ice went out of favor because cold is not healing. The inflammation is part of your body's natural healing process and cold can slow that down. Don't feel too bad about using cold/ice though, as cold can be used when necessary to keep pain and swelling/inflammation from getting out of hand. Cold can reduce pain by numbing the nerves and thus is great for temporary pain control. You don't want so much cold that you damage your skin, so use something that isn't too cold. Or, when using ice directly, keep the ice moving and stop once the region feels numb. A direct ice treatment can be helpful for temporary relief when injured or to break the pain-cycle in a chronic pain syndrome. Ice as it melts can get slippery. One way to prepare ice for direct use is to freeze water in a paper cup and then peel half the cup away to reveal the ice. You could use a water popsicle too, if you have at-home popsicle molds. Once you are going to apply the ice to the skin, you need to keep it moving, either back and forth or in circles. There is an acronym: CBAN. It represents the stages of cold treatment: cold, burning, achiness, and then numbness. As soon as you hit numbness, stop. It should take about 2-5 minutes.

Contrast therapy uses both hot and cold. People on the internet argue about how long you should use each before switching. Some say 2 min, some 5 min, and others 10 min. I've been splitting the difference and telling people about 5 minutes each for 2 cycles with a short break between switching to allow the skin temperature to equalize. I see contrast therapy as having 2 advantages. Firstly, it gives you a chance to try both so you can get a feel if either is particularly relieving so that you can use that one exclusively in the future if shorter on time. Secondly, the cold drives fluid away from the area and heat brings fluid towards the area. This is thought to pump fluid in and out. Some patients have reported feeling the pain draining out of the region. I recommend this in particular for the pain caused by ischemic compression that some feel the day after treatment.

Whole body treatments such as a sauna for heat or whole-body cryotherapy for cold may have additional effects in addition to the local effects described. The research is all over the place, though. Sauna therapy has had the most research. For at least some types of chronic pain, it offers immediate relief and the benefits might be long lasting.[72,73] For whole-body cryotherapy, which is much newer, the research is lacking but there are some positive findings.[74,75] I've heard mixed reviews and experiences from patients: nothing bad, but some said it didn't seem to have a lasting impact. Maybe it depends on the source/type of the pain—central sensitization, muscle knots, etc.

---

[72] Hussain J, Cohen M. Clinical Effects of Regular Dry Sauna Bathing: A Systematic Review. *Evid Based Complement Alternat Med.* 2018;2018:1857413. doi:10.1155/2018/1857413

[73] Cho EH, Kim NH, Kim HC, Yang YH, Kim J, Hwang B. Dry sauna therapy is beneficial for patients with low back pain. *Anesth Pain Med (Seoul).* 2019;14(4):474-479. doi:10.17085/apm.2019.14.4.474

[74] Garcia C, Karri J, Zacharias NA, Abd-Elsayed A. Use of Cryotherapy for Managing Chronic Pain: An Evidence-Based Narrative. *Pain Ther.* 2021;10(1):81-100. doi:10.1007/s40122-020-00225-w

[75] Salas-Fraire O, Rivera-Pérez JA, Guevara-Neri NP, et al. Efficacy of whole-body cryotherapy in the treatment of chronic low back pain: Quasi-experimental study. *J Orthop Sci.* 2023;28(1):112-116. doi:10.1016/j.jos.2021.10.006

Ischemic Compression

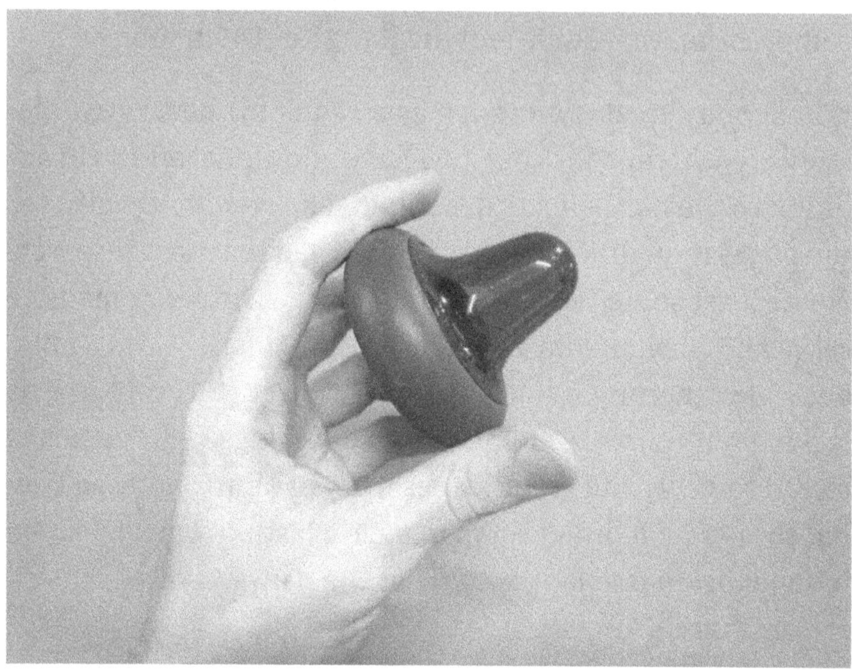

Ischemic compression is a very effective way of treating myofascial trigger points and can eliminate them in a single treatment. Ischemia is depriving tissue of blood so the idea behind ischemic compression is to deprive the muscle knot of blood through compression. I like to think of it as punishing the muscle knot until it behaves itself, "No blood for you until you leave this poor woman/man alone!" You have to push right in the center of the knot. If you are to the side, the muscle fibers might pull on the knot triggering the pain but the knot won't go away because you aren't squishing the source of the problem. There are trigger point tools that aid in compressing the knots but your knuckles or the handle of a spoon/screwdriver/wrench can work just as well in a pinch. When you compress the knot, you should feel it recreate the pain. In particular, you may feel the pain spread. This spreading can be very confusing as the location of the muscle knot and the location of the pain can be quite different: muscle knots in the glutes (butt region) can refer down the leg, muscle knots in the shoulders can refer to above the eye, or muscle knots on the scapula (shoulder blade) can refer to the front of the shoulder and down the arm. You can visit triggerpoints.net for a map to get an idea of where they could be or refer to the rest of this book as I'll point out some of the more common ones.

Once you have identified the point, the treatment is as follows:

- You compress the MFTP until pain reaches about a 5/10.

- Within 60 seconds, the pain should drop if you are in the right place and have the right diagnosis.

- Once the pain drops, increase the pressure until pain goes back to 5/10.

- Within 30 seconds, the pain should drop again.

- Increase the pressure again repeating the cycle until the pain stops dropping, it feels like you are just pushing into the bone, or the patient says they only feel pressure.

- Once you release, they should be able to immediately feel a difference.

- Recheck next to where you were working and in the general area to see if there are more spots to treat, particularly if there was still some pain in the last phase of the treatment.

- Repeat the process, if necessary, on subsequent days. You may skip a day if the area is a bit throbbing/achy from treatment the day before.

This is a very safe treatment and can be self-done provided you can find the point. It is unlikely to result in any bruising. The muscle knots are full of chemical messengers for pain and inflammation, so by getting rid of the muscle knot, these chemicals are released and they may interact with the surrounding tissue. Some people report feeling a throbbing, achy pain that starts that evening or the next day, which normally clears up in 24 hours.

The only possible worry for an amateur for doing something like this is confusing a muscle knot with a deep vein thrombosis (blood clot in the leg which can present as a tender band in the calf). A deep vein thrombosis (DVT) occurs typically with lack of movement and is typically post-surgical, and typically the leg is swollen and red. Massaging or compressing the deep vein thrombosis can dislodge the thrombosis (a blood clot/clump) which can travel to the lungs and cause a pulmonary embolism (lung blood flow blockage). On a relatively normal, non-swollen leg and anywhere else in the body, the technique is very safe.

Acupuncture/Dry Needling

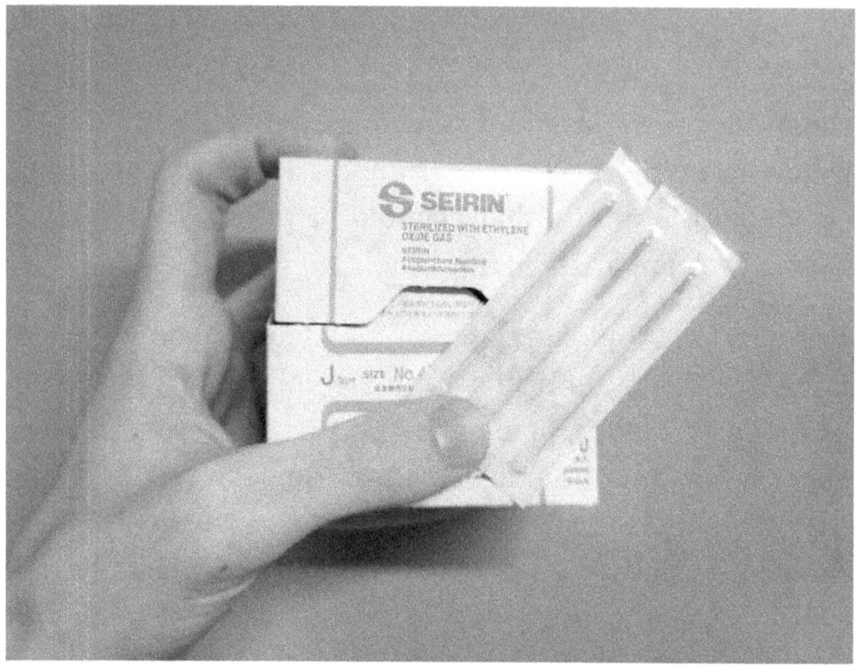

Dry needling is the term used when you use a needle without injecting anything. The term is used more when using acupuncture needles to relax tight muscles or resolve muscle knots. The term is most commonly used by physiotherapists and chiropractors. Acupuncture refers to putting needles at the acupuncture points along the meridians. Chiropractors or physiotherapists may also use these points, but acupuncturists are known for this. Similarly, acupuncturists may deviate from the meridians and points to treat the muscles directly like the other practitioners.

Acupuncture is surprisingly pain free. The typical needles are single use and are very thin—so thin that you can place an acupuncture needle within the tube of a typical injection needle. Unlike an injection needle that cuts a hole into the skin, the acupuncture needle hardly leaves a trace. It is rare for there to be even a drop of blood and it can be very challenging to see where the needle was. When done well, the needle should be painless. You might feel a jolt as the needle punctures the skin and the muscle might twitch, but you should feel nothing or a sense of pressure once the needle is settled. The sense of pressure is the ideal scenario as that is indicative of hitting a real good spot where the needle will have a significant effect. It may be so comfortable that some patients drool or fall asleep full of needles.

It has been fairly well established that acupuncture treatments help with pain, which is why some insurance companies cover acupuncture (although you might need a referral from an MD).[76] The exact mechanism isn't understood and the quality of research is a little rocky as, similar to exercise and muscle work, how do you have a proper placebo to compare with and who is going to pay for this research?[77,78]

Dry needling is one of the better ways of treating nasty muscle knots (myofascial trigger points, MFTPs).[79] In some

[76] Xiang A, Cheng K, Shen X, Xu P, Liu S. The Immediate Analgesic Effect of Acupuncture for Pain: A Systematic Review and Meta-Analysis. *Evid Based Complement Alternat Med.* 2017;2017:3837194. doi:10.1155/2017/3837194

[77] Paley CA, Johnson MI. Acupuncture for the Relief of Chronic Pain: A Synthesis of Systematic Reviews. *Medicina (Kaunas).* 2019;56(1):6. Published 2019 Dec 24. doi:10.3390/medicina56010006

[78] Chys M, De Meulemeester K, De Greef I, et al. Clinical Effectiveness of Dry Needling in Patients with Musculoskeletal Pain-An Umbrella Review. *J Clin Med.* 2023;12(3):1205. Published 2023 Feb 2. doi:10.3390/jcm12031205

[79] Navarro-Santana MJ, Sanchez-Infante J, Fernández-de-las-Peñas C, Cleland JA, Martín-Casas P, Plaza-Manzano G. Effectiveness of Dry Needling for Myo-

studies, dry needling was superior to ischemic compression, but in other studies, the results were reversed. In my clinical experimentation with patients, I found needling was more effective in the arms and legs but slightly less effective than compression in the shoulders, neck, and hips. Needling is very effective for achy, tight, ropy muscles, often much more effective than pin-and-stretch or massage.

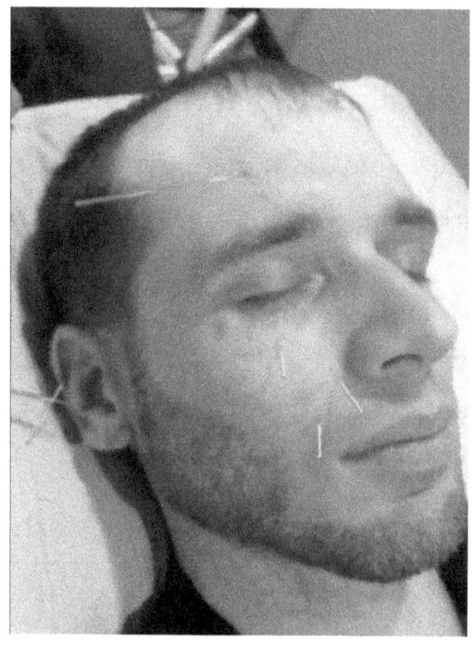

One of the proposed mechanisms for the changes caused by the needles is it causes changes in local blood flow. This is visible in those with fair skin. I can often see slowly enlarging pink circles as the area of increased blood flow expands as the needle does its thing.

---

fascial Trigger Points Associated with Neck Pain Symptoms: An Updated Systematic Review and Meta-Analysis. *Journal of Clinical Medicine.* 2020; 9(10):3300. https://doi.org/10.3390/jcm9103300

Needling may help with tendinosis. The research on it isn't great, but it does seem to help.[80] I think even a single acupuncture needle may help through its ability to alter local blood flow. If you start poking the needle around with the intent of making holes in the tendon, it can be called fenestration (see the next section). Fenestration can be done with acupuncture needles or with larger needles to cause larger holes.

Fenestration

This is a treatment for tendinosis. Recall that tendinosis is a chronically painful and sickly tendon. The body's upkeep is either insufficient and/or the wear and tear is too high. Eliminating the increased wear-and tear might be easily done by taking a break from playing tennis (tennis elbow) but how do you get the body to improve its upkeep and rebuild the tendon properly? What if we damage the tendon on purpose? Then the body has to fix it! This sounds extreme, and it is, but tendinosis can be very persistent. They take a very thick needle and poke holes in the tendon so it looks like Swiss cheese. This procedure can be done with a local anesthetic, and typically by a medical doctor. You may be leaving with your arm in a sling or on crutches. Gentler versions of fenestration can be done with smaller, acupuncture needles, typically by an acupuncturist, physiotherapist, or chiropractor. Both the more extreme version and the

---

[80] Boström, K., Mæhlum, S., Cvancarova Småstuen, M. et al. Clinical comparative effectiveness of acupuncture versus manual therapy treatment of lateral epicondylitis: feasibility randomized clinical trial. *Pilot Feasibility Stud* 5, 110 (2019). https://doi.org/10.1186/s40814-019-0490-x

gentler acupuncture/dry needling version have reasonably good results.[81]

PRP, Prolotherapy (dextrose), and Stem Cells

PRP, prolotherapy, and stem cells are all types of injections that aim to improve your body's natural healing. These are low risk treatments, so I recommend them to those with particularly stubborn problems or, in the case of stem cells, those with the money for it. Worst case is they don't help your chronic problem.

PRP stands for Platelet-Rich-Protein injection. Some of your own blood is removed, then put into a centrifuge to isolate the "good stuff," the stuff your body uses for repair. Then this is injected into the region with the pain/damage such as with a tendinosis.[82] Those with arthritis pain may benefit from PRP injections in or around their joints (keep in mind that your pain might not be related to the arthritis). The injections in most studies seem to reduce pain, improve function, and it may reduce the rate of cartilage thinning.[83] For

---

[81] Stoychev V, Finestone AS, Kalichman L. Dry Needling as a Treatment Modality for Tendinopathy: a Narrative Review. *Curr Rev Musculoskelet Med.* 2020;13(1):133-140. doi:10.1007/s12178-020-09608-0

[82] Miller LE, Parrish WR, Roides B, *et al.* Efficacy of platelet-rich plasma injections for symptomatic tendinopathy: systematic review and meta-analysis of randomised injection-controlled trials. *BMJ Open Sport & Exercise Medicine* 2017;3:e000237. doi: 10.1136/bmjsem-2017-000237

[83] Rodríguez-Merchán EC. Intra-Articular Platelet-Rich Plasma Injections in Knee Osteoarthritis: A Review of Their Current Molecular Mechanisms of Action and Their Degree of Efficacy. *Int J Mol Sci.* 2022;23(3):1301. Published 2022 Jan 24. doi:10.3390/ijms23031301

many conditions like plantar fasciitis/fasciosis and TMJ pain, PRP seems to be superior to cortisone injections without the damage that cortisone can cause.[84,85]

Prolotherapy is typically an injection of dextrose into the painful and/or damaged tissue such as with a tendinosis. While every doctor might use a slightly different concoction, the most typical ingredient is dextrose. Dextrose is a form of glucose, a sugar. The thought is that the injection of sugar straight into the painful tissue irritates it and causes an acute inflammatory reaction which can kick-start the body to repair the problem area. I have heard from those with personal experience that it can be painful for a few days after treatment (which is why some docs combine the dextrose with things like pain relievers/anesthetics). I've heard of it resolving a chronic problem that had bothered them for years and did not resolve with soft tissue work and exercises. A systematic review on prolotherapy for chronic pain concluded that prolotherapy was an effective treatment for tendinopathies (tendon issues), spine/pelvic ligament issues, and for knee/finger osteoarthritis.[86]

[84] Hohmann E, Tetsworth K, Glatt V. Platelet-Rich Plasma Versus Corticosteroids for the Treatment of Plantar Fasciitis: A Systematic Review and Meta-analysis. *Am J Sports Med.* 2021;49(5):1381-1393. doi:10.1177/0363546520937293

[85] Gokçe Kutuk S, Gökçe G, Arslan M, Özkan Y, Kütük M, Kursat Arikan O. Clinical and Radiological Comparison of Effects of Platelet-Rich Plasma, Hyaluronic Acid, and Corticosteroid Injections on Temporomandibular Joint Osteoarthritis. *J Craniofac Surg.* 2019;30(4):1144-1148. doi:10.1097/SCS.0000000000005211

[86] Hauser RA, Lackner JB, Steilen-Matias D, Harris DK. A Systematic Review of Dextrose Prolotherapy for Chronic Musculoskeletal Pain. *Clin Med Insights*

Stem cells are still in a more experimental stage. I would consider it safe, but the FDA is unconvinced due to the small volume of research. How effective it is for each possible condition definitely hasn't been well established as we mostly just have case studies to go on. The clinic I worked in (DVC STEM) offers stem cell treatment for about $25,000 USD. Some of the rich are using it for anti-aging and for nagging aches. Some individuals treat this as a last resort, having tried everything else. Maybe their condition is so severe that they are desperate. There are two types of stem cells: ones removed from your own body with limited ability to differentiate into other cells and fresh young stem cells (mesenchymal cells) that can turn into any cell in the body. The young stem cells are obviously the more expensive and seen as the better option. Mesenchymal stem cells are a popular option for nerve pain, particularly for neurodegenerative conditions, neuropathy from chemotherapy, brain damage from stroke, etc. as they can replace nerve cells and promote nerve growth.[87,88] Response to treatment can be good, but not all patients experience a benefit and how much of a benefit is variable. I wonder if the placebo effect could be impacting results. That being said, I have seen it

---

Arthritis Musculoskelet Disord. 2016;9:139-159. Published 2016 Jul 7. doi:10.4137/CMAMD.S39160

[87] Ji XL, Ma L, Zhou WH, Xiong M. Narrative review of stem cell therapy for ischemic brain injury. *Transl Pediatr.* 2021;10(2):435-445. doi:10.21037/tp-20-262

[88] Fortino VR, Pelaez D, Cheung HS. Concise review: stem cell therapies for neuropathic pain. *Stem Cells Transl Med.* 2013;2(5):394-399. doi:10.5966/sctm.2012-0122

work! I have personally seen nagging pain go away and I've seen people with no sensation regain some.

Steroid Injections (Cortisone)

Cortisone and other steroids are strong anti-inflammatories. They can provide short term pain relief. They can break down and destroy scar tissue… but also healthy tissue. Since they can damage tissue like tendons they should be used cautiously. They are best injected with ultrasound imaging guidance. See the earlier section of this book on "Do Cortisone Injections Help?" for more information.

Anesthetic/Nerve Blocks

Anesthetic injections or nerve blocks can be useful for very short-term relief and to positively identify a pain generator.[89] With X-rays and MRIs, you can identify structural issues, but how do you know whether these structural issues are causing pain or not? Lots of things look bad on MRI or X-ray, but which ones, if any, are the culprit. Injecting an anesthetic can let you identify the structure/region causing some of your pain if it provides some relief. It is best injected with imaging guidance. The placebo effect can help as well. Just the fact you are getting an injection can help with

---

[89] Atluri S, Datta S, Falco FJ, Lee M. Systematic review of diagnostic utility and therapeutic effectiveness of thoracic facet joint interventions. *Pain Physician.* 2008;11(5):611-629.

the pain. Although possibly not as bad as cortisone, anesthetics are toxic to cartilage cells so it should be used prudently if joints are involved.[90]

Anesthetics/nerve blocks can lead to long term relief because they can let you start moving/exercising, and they give you a break from the pain which can help combat central sensitization.

Nerve Ablation

From reading this book, you should have a sense of the difficulty in finding the source of someone's pain. **If** the exact nerve that is responsible for setting off the pain system can be identified through a nerve block, then a doctor could destroy that nerve for a more permanent solution. This nerve destruction is sometimes called radiofrequency ablation, and they use radio waves to create concentrated heat to burn the nerve. This is a minimally invasive procedure and done with imaging guidance to make sure they are in the right area.

The nerve may grow back in 6 to 9 months. If there was overlapping pain from other structures, some pain may persist. Some central sensitization, fear of movement, etc. might still need to be worked on. The downsides are it might not work and there is a rare chance of increased pain or infection. The success rate in one study in the low back was

[90] Gulihar A, Robati S, Twaij H, Salih A, Taylor GJ. Articular cartilage and local anaesthetic: A systematic review of the current literature. *J Orthop.* 2015;12(Suppl 2):S200-S210. Published 2015 Oct 31. doi:10.1016/j.jor.2015.10.005

76% at 7–21 days after the denervation, 32% at 6 months, and 22% at 1 year.[91] They found that those with depression were less likely to respond well to treatment.

Joint Aspiration

Aspirations are an option for fluid in a cyst, bursa, or joint. In an aspiration, they pull out the excess fluid. In some cases, this can resolve issues and in others this may only provide temporary relief. Aspirations can be done without ultrasound guidance, but some, like synovial/ganglion cysts benefit from visualization where the physician can see where the cyst is connected to the joint and they can try to scar it up the connection to prevent the cyst from returning. Ganglion cysts can be removed entirely instead of being aspirated as another option more specific to that type of cyst.

Pin-and-stretch and ART

This is a type of muscle relaxation technique for tight and achy muscles. First, you shorten the muscle, then push on the muscle, then move the limb/body to stretch the muscle while you have maintained the pressure. Take off pressure, then repeat. Some people hold the stretch for a protracted amount of time, but I find a few rounds of about 5-6 seconds seems to do the trick. A similar strategy can be employed to break up scar tissue and fascial adhesions causing reduced

---

[91] Streitberger K, Müller T, Eichenberger U, Trelle S, Curatolo M. Factors determining the success of radiofrequency denervation in lumbar facet joint pain: a prospective study. *Eur Spine J.* 2011;20(12):2160-2165. doi:10.1007/s00586-011-1891-6

movement, tightness, pinching, or pulling. You grab and hold down the tight spot as the limb/body is moved to pull things free.

There is a common certification called Active Release Techniques (ART) which involves this style of treatment. Pin-and-stretch and ART both require an excellent visualization of the anatomy and the action of each muscle.

Fascial Adhesion Release

This isn't an official named treatment technique, but I chose this term to describe a class of techniques that allow tissue to move freely if they have been bound up by adhesions sticking the tissue together from inactivity or post-injury. If the skin isn't gliding in all directions, I sometimes thrust it in the direction it won't move to release it. Skin rolling and slide cupping can work by lifting the skin away from the muscles, breaking any painful and limiting adhesions. If the muscles are stuck to one another, grabbing/isolating the muscle and vigorously pushing/shaking it can release adhesions (one version of this is called "rolfing"). Pin-and-stretch/ART can also release adhesions and are particularly useful if you know which structure is limiting motion.

Cross-friction (Deep-friction Massage)

Cross-friction (deep-friction) massage is similar to some of the previous techniques because it can be used to break up adhesions/scar tissue, but it has other applications as well. The treatment is done by first identifying a painful structure, then grinding/rubbing/moving the structure perpendicular to the direction of fibers. This is done deeply and vigorously and can be 9/10 on the pain scale. This causes increased blood flow, can break-up or prevent adhesions, and can encourage fibers to rebuild properly. In the healing stages of a ligament sprain or tendon tear, the body lays down a patch of disorganized tissue. Once that is done, it goes through and remodels it. Cross-friction massage can help the remodeling process.

A tendinosis is like an unfinished remodeling phase. The tendon just hasn't healed to full health. Similarly, ankle pain from an old injury might be a patch of disorganized tissue that was never remodeled. Cross-friction can be the key to making progress on stubborn ligament and tendon pain.[92,93]

[92] Joseph MF, Taft K, Moskwa M, Denegar CR. Deep Friction Massage to Treat Tendinopathy: A Systematic Review of a Classic Treatment in the Face of a New Paradigm of Understanding. *Journal of Sport Rehabilitation.* 2012;21(4):343-353. doi:10.1123/jsr.21.4.343

[93] Yi R, Bratchenko WW, Tan V. Deep Friction Massage Versus Steroid Injection in the Treatment of Lateral Epicondylitis. *Hand* (N Y). 2018;13(1):56-59. doi:10.1177/1558944717692088

Instrument Assisted Soft Tissue Mobilization (Gua Sha, Graston, RockBlades, etc.)

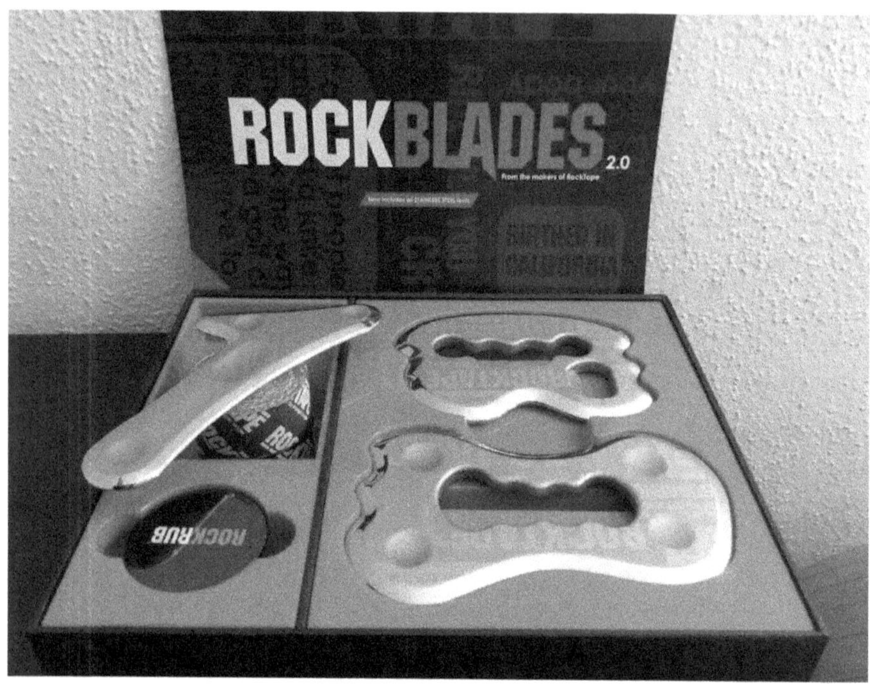

Instrument Assisted Soft Tissue Mobilization (IASTM) involves using a jade, plastic, or steel tool to aid in tissue treatment. The other soft tissue treatments covered in this section can often be aided with a tool to make the treatment more effective and/or to help protect the practitioner's fingers/hands. The most common technique is similar to cross friction massage because the goal is to break adhesions/scar tissue and increase local blood flow. With a massage oil or lubricant, the tool is slid over the tissue, the practitioner feels for regions of where the tool's movement is bumpy and then goes over that region more vigorously until it feels smoother. While it is typical for the region to be a bit red afterwards, if your skin looks like bacon, the practitioner was a bit too aggressive. Some have the belief that the more redness and blood the better, but the problem is under the skin so there is no need to damage the skin.

The tools can be combined with other techniques that typically use hands/fingers. A muscle stripping massage for muscle relaxation can be done with the tools: you slowly press and follow the muscle along its path. This technique is typically done on the skin with massage oil, but it can be done through clothing fairly effectively. Cross friction massage and skin mobilization can be done with the tool as well. In this case, do without the use of massage oil because you don't want the tool to slide on the skin.

The tool can be used to help proprioception by rubbing it gently and quickly along the skin, often combined with joint movement. The thought is that the extra skin stimulation helps the brain figure out what the joint is doing allowing the brain to relearn control more effectively. If the skin is abnormally sensitive to touch due to central sensitization, using very light pressure with a hand, steel tool, hair brush, etc. can help return the pain threshold to normal.

Cupping

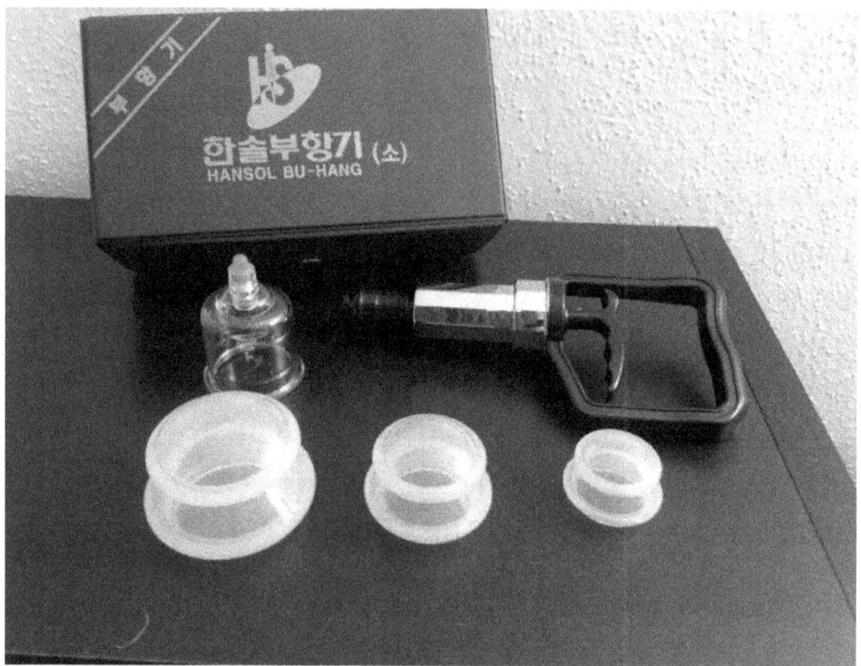

Cupping uses suction to lift the skin and is believed to have been done for thousands of years.[94] Historically, it might have been for pulling out toxins and impurities from the body, whereas now it is more used for fascial manipulation or for lymphatic drainage. Some people find cupping sessions profoundly relaxing, both mentally and physically. There are various versions of the cups and various strategies have been used throughout the years. You can still find the full gamut of cupping usage today.

---

[94] Qureshi NA, Ali GI, Abushanab TS, et al. History of cupping (Hijama): a narrative review of literature. *J Integr Med.* 2017;15(3):172-181. doi:10.1016/S2095-4964(17)60339-X

The modern usage of cupping involves glass, plastic, or silicone cups. The suction is created with a hand pump, by deforming the silicone, or by an attached vacuum pump machine. The purpose is not to generate purple circular bruises but to release fascial restrictions or to aid in lymphatic drainage (see the lymphatic massage section). If the skin isn't sliding over the muscles well, this can lead to a pulling sensation or even a sharp pain. I tend to use the moving/sliding cupping technique where I slide the cup along the skin over the restricted area (using lotion/oil) or I'll place the cup statically on the skin and have them move their limb. If there is no problem, then this is very comfortable, but the worse the restriction is, the more difficult it will be for the cup to lift the skin, and the more painful it will be as the cup breaks the adhesions. This strategy can be done with the fingers in which case it is called skin rolling, but the cups make it soooo much easier. I find the silicone cups work best for this. Fascial cupping is most often done by chiropractors and physiotherapists. While fascial or lymphatic work might only require one or two cups, a more traditional cupping session may use a dozen or more cups. Traditionally you'll find glass, plastic, or even horns used. The suction may be created by a pump but may also be created through fire (fire cupping). The practitioner may even cut the skin before applying the cups to cause bleeding (bleed out the bad stuff... right?) and this is called "wet cupping." Don't let me scare you with the blood. Places that do cupping sessions will be more than happy to do "dry cupping" instead of "wet cupping" on request. More traditional cupping sessions are more likely to be done by an acupuncturist or a massage therapist.

The plastic cupping kits or silicone cups are relatively cheap at $20-$50, and with some common sense, are usable by amateurs. Cupping might be an appropriate date night activity with your partner.

Lymphatic Massage

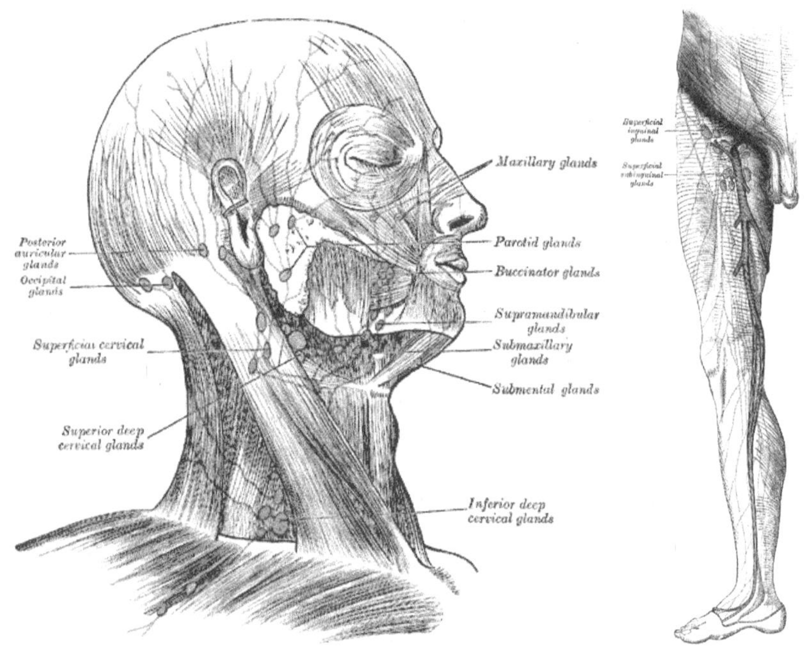

A lymphatic massage attempts to aid the flow of lymph fluid through the body. But... What the heck is lymph fluid? Most people have heard of lymph nodes and are aware that if they are enlarged it can be a sign of infection/sickness/cancer but don't learn anything beyond that.

Let's do a quick lesson on the lymphatic system. The role of the lymphatic system is to control the amount of fluid in our tissues and to monitor for infections. Most people know about the arteries (carrying fresh oxygenated blood) and the veins (carrying deoxygenated blood), but did you know that we have a separate set of vessels throughout our body? These vessels do not have a pump like the heart, so these lymph vessels have one-way valves inside them. When the vessel is squished (by pressing on the skin or contracting a muscle) that squeezes the fluid along the path. What fluid is it and where does it come from? When your blood drops off nutrients and oxygen and then picks up carbon dioxide and chemicals to be expelled, some fluid is lost to the tissue. The lymphatic system picks up the extra fluid that doesn't make its way to the veins. When you are injured, the area becomes inflamed and fluid piles up. The lymphatic system is what ultimately will take all that extra fluid away. The lymph nodes are the sentinels of the body. Your body has immune cells there to check the fluid for infections. Ultimately the fluid slowly makes its way to just above the heart where it is dumped into the blood system.

Since the lymphatic fluid doesn't move on its own, you have to move your body for the system to work. You can help the fluid along by purposefully and repeatedly pumping fluid through the vessels with gentle pressure and sweeping movements (called a manual lymphatic massage). Most vessels are just under the skin, so you don't need too much pressure. Slide cupping works well. A vacuum lymphatic massage involves using a vacuum pump and a glass cup to accelerate lymphatic fluid drainage.

In a perfect world, everyone would receive multiple lymphatic massage sessions after any major surgery as all that extra fluid needs to get through the lymphatic system, and this can be made worse by lack of movement post-surgery.

If you are older and have had heavy swollen limbs since an injury or surgery, maybe your body was never able to clear out the extra fluid. A couple lymphatic massage sessions can help resolve this type of chronic swelling. I'm not an expert at it, but after speaking to an expert (Maja Pesic), she gets better results with vacuum suction lymphatic drainage in comparison to the manual (hand) version. Elevation combined with contracting your muscles can help, such as elevating your legs while doing calf exercises could help with lymphatic drainage out of the ankles.

Lymphatic drainage massages are typically done by a massage therapist or a physiotherapist. They might have CLT (certified lymphedema therapist) next to their name, indicating additional training.

Chiropractic Adjustments (joint manipulations/mobilizations)

What is a chiropractic adjustment/manipulation?

A chiropractic adjustment or a chiropractic joint manipulation is a quick thrust to a joint for pain relief and/or to restore proper motion/symmetry. The "pop" sound isn't necessary to receive a benefit, but some patients expect it and some chiropractors choose adjustments that result in loud pops. The benefit comes from the quickness of the movement which can result in a reflex relaxation of the nearby muscles.[95] The loud popping adjustments are also called grade 5 joint mobilizations. The other grades of joint mobilization are less extreme and may also be effective at restoring proper motion. The quickness of a chiropractic adjustment seems to have a nervous system impact and may help people's pain via the central nervous system.[96] Chiropractors aren't the only ones doing chiropractic adjustments anymore. They are often taught to osteopaths and physiotherapists as well. They have an established track record of being safe and effective, so it only makes sense for the other professions to want to use them as well to help their patients. By "effective," I want to be clear that it isn't effective for everything, and the effects can be short lived. Sometimes it can be the miracle treatment where the person's problem instantly goes away (mild stiffness, most rib pain, and some pelvic pain).

Does the chiropractor have to crack/pop my spine?

No. There are alternative ways of restoring segmental motion in the spine that do not involve creating a pop/crack. The pop/crack should not be the ultimate goal of the chiropractor. The main goal of the chiropractor, osteopath, or physiotherapist is often to eliminate asymmetries, reduce pain, and restore proper motion. There are handheld devices which deliver an impulse right where the chiropractor wants. The most common one is called an activator tool or

---

[95] Pickar JG, Bolton PS. Spinal manipulative therapy and somatosensory activation. *J Electromyogr Kinesiol.* 2012;22(5):785-794. doi:10.1016/j.jelekin.2012.01.015

[96] Pickar JG. Neurophysiological effects of spinal manipulation. *Spine J.* 2002;2(5):357-371. doi:10.1016/s1529-9430(02)00400-x

"clicker." The other option is just a gentle mobilization of the joint (often combined with a muscle relaxation technique like MET or a stretch). This gentle mobilization just involves applying a gentle force to the joint, either with movement or rhythmically back and force. Sometimes, though, the standard high velocity low amplitude (HVLA) chiropractic adjustment is the most effective and quickest way to restore motion. You can request your health practitioner to use alternative methods first. For myself, I respond well to and prefer the "clicker" or gentle mobilization in my neck but for my mid back, I find HVLA works best there. Every person's body is different.

Are chiropractic adjustments safe?

The short answer is yes. Are there adverse events that occur? Yes, but so rare I wouldn't be worried about it. I'd be more worried about taking ibuprofen than a chiropractic adjustment as chance of a more severe adverse event is about 3 in a million for a chiropractic adjustment,[97] but 100,000 people per year go to the emergency room and 10,000-20,000/year die from ibuprofen in the US.[98] The severe adverse event for chiropractic adjustments is typically a rib fracture in an osteoporotic woman which is a risk you can easily understand if someone is using a quick thrust to

---

[97] Chu, E.CP., Trager, R.J., Lee, L.YK. et al. A retrospective analysis of the incidence of severe adverse events among recipients of chiropractic spinal manipulative therapy. *Sci Rep 13*, 1254 (2023). https://doi.org/10.1038/s41598-023-28520-4

[98] Singh G. Recent considerations in nonsteroidal anti-inflammatory drug gastropathy. *Am J Med*. 1998;105(1B):31S-38S. doi:10.1016/s0002-9343(98)00072-2

loosen a rib joint and/or mid back joint. There are very severe cervical artery related strokes or dissections (tears of the artery) but those may have happened anyway or may have started before seeing the chiropractor as, statistically, people who visit chiropractors are not more likely to have these artery events.[99] The symptoms of these events could be a headache with neck pain, which is a typical reason for people to seek out a chiropractor. Also, manipulations don't cause more stress on the artery than normal full neck rotations.[100] A diseased artery event may be triggered by turning the head while driving, putting away the dishes, or with a chiropractor turning your neck, but we aren't scared of shoulder checking the way some people are scared of their neck being cracked.

[99] Whedon, J.M., Petersen, C.L., Li, Z. et al. Association between cervical artery dissection and spinal manipulative therapy –a medicare claims analysis. *BMC Geriatr* 22, 917 (2022). https://doi.org/10.1186/s12877-022-03495-5

[100] Symons B, Herzog W. Cervical artery dissection: a biomechanical perspective. *J Can Chiropr Assoc.* 2013;57(4):276-278.

Activator

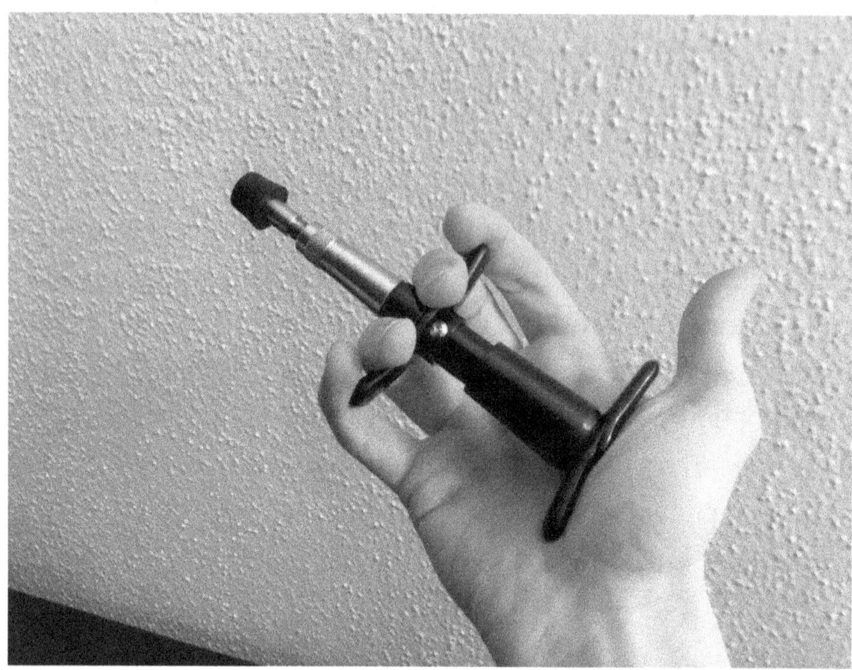

The activator is a tool which provides a quick thrust but it is not forceful enough to cause a cracking/popping sound. The current theory for why chiropractic adjustments work has to do more with the quick stretch rather than the cracking sound. There is a stretch receptor (Golgi tendon apparatus) in muscles that, if you stretch it fast enough, can cause reflexive relaxation. If the activator tool can cause that stretch then you can get the same benefit as the "crack."

Many people are apprehensive about having their neck cracked/adjusted, so the activator tool is a convenient way of treating them without having their neck cracked. The initial tool is out of patent so you can buy a cheaper version of the original called a "chiropractic adjustment tool" (CAT). Many chiropractors call it the "clicker." There are electric versions of it as well.

There is also an "activator technique system." The chiropractic profession loves their named technique systems (Logan, Gonstead, activator, Webster, etc.). Not only is it a treatment, but also an evaluation system. In this case, by looking at the length of your legs, they guess as to what spots in your spine are your issues. I am not trained in the activator technique system, but having talked to those who have taken it, the algorithm can be fairly accurate and it is fast. But the two I talked to still planned to evaluate the joints the old-fashioned way. Most chiropractors who say they use the activator refer to the tool and not the technique system.

Massage Therapy / Muscle Massagers (percussion massagers)

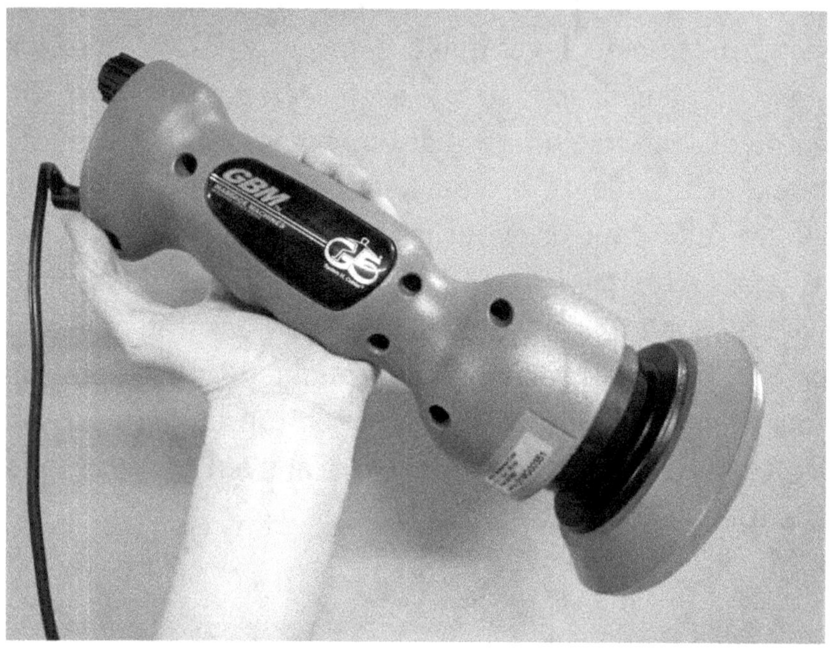

I'm lumping massage therapy in with electronic massagers because I believe their mechanisms and effectiveness are similar. Massage therapists are typically trained in Swedish massage. They may have learned other specialized techniques, but that isn't necessarily the case. The electric massagers vibrate/oscillate to shake or "punch" the tissue repeatedly. They often have different intensity settings and multiple attachments. Both styles can be more intense or less intense.

Both massagers are good for releasing muscle tension and providing short term pain relief. If the body wants those muscles to stay tight, they might tighten back up quickly. More aggressive massager settings or more aggressive manual massage can break up scar tissue and adhesions. The skin contact and tissue manipulation can help with central sensitization/fibromyalgia, by helping the nervous system to relax.[101] I find higher, buzzier, settings are better for distracting the nervous system and I found the slower, deeper, settings better for muscle relaxation. Massage is not very good at relieving nasty, painful muscle knots. The repeated grinding of a masseuse can be very painful with only short term and/or partial relief. I was so excited that my very expensive, professional grade G5 massager had a recommended myofascial trigger point treatment protocol. To their credit, it did work 50% of the time, but ischemic compression works 100% of the time. Get rid of muscle knots first before a deep-tissue-type massage to have a more enjoyable experience.

Webster Technique

Since many chiropractors only do joint manipulations, it is sometimes helpful to know names of techniques that involve muscles when searching for a chiropractor. Dr. Webster, based on just a couple of pregnant patients, found that there were some patterns of asymmetry and muscle/ligament tightness for the pelvis. He came up with a condensed way of quickly evaluating the nature of the pattern (which side) and an efficient minimal treatment protocol of just a

---

[101] Li Y-h, Wang F-y, Feng C-q, Yang X-f, Sun Y-h (2014) Massage Therapy for Fibromyalgia: A Systematic Review and Meta-Analysis of Randomized Controlled Trials. PLoS ONE 9(2): e89304. https://doi.org/10.1371/journal.pone.0089304

few key structures that fits well in the medium to high volume chiropractic practice. While it was designed for pregnant mothers, it can be beneficial to those with any pelvic asymmetry/pain. While I did do the Webster Technique training, I personally don't follow the exact protocol.

Cranial Techniques

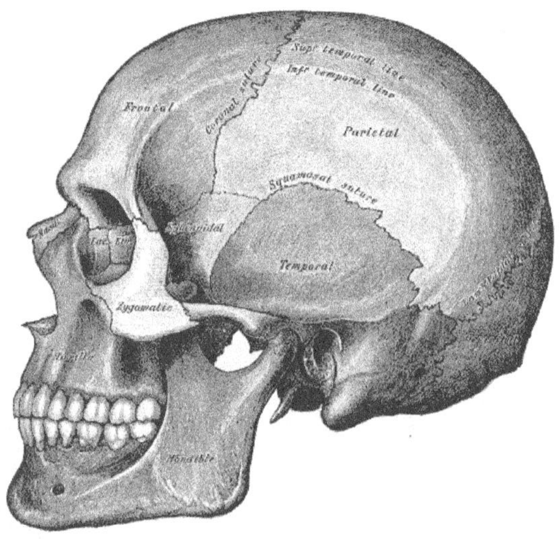

Cranial techniques are techniques that involve applying pressure to the skull and may be performed by osteopaths, chiropractors, or massage therapists. Historically, this was done to attempt to move, loosen, and/or shift the cranial bones. Some of the claimed benefits involving improved cognition and memory are attributed to increased cerebral spinal fluid flow from increased cranial bone mobility.[102] Cerebral spinal fluid flow is still an active area of research, but none of the theories being investigated by the medical

---

[102] https://www.cranialtherapycentre.com/a-beginners-guide-to-craniosacral-therapy/

     BRANDON RAMAKKO

community involve cranial bones.[103] The joints of the skull are fibrous joints and eventually ossify. These are not mobile joints, and chiropractors/osteopaths advertising moving these bones are mocked in the medical community.[104]

That being said, these techniques can be profoundly relaxing, and I've found them helpful with very stubborn headaches and sinus congestion. It can "feel" as though the bones are moving. Who cares why it works if it helps! The skull is wrapped in layers of fascia and tissue which I think is the mechanism why these techniques can be effective. In fact, these layers have been linked to stubborn post-concussion headaches.[105] Certain acupressure points related to the sinuses are typically used with cranial techniques, and they can provide temporary relief of sinus congestion in some individuals (I often teach these to my patients if they are relieving).

---

[103] Wichmann TO, Damkier HH and Pedersen M (2022) A Brief Overview of the Cerebrospinal Fluid System and Its Implications for Brain and Spinal Cord Diseases. *Front. Hum. Neurosci.* 15:737217. doi: 10.3389/fnhum.2021.737217

[104] Hartman SE. Cranial osteopathy: its fate seems clear. *Chiropr Osteopat.* 2006;14:10. Published 2006 Jun 8. doi:10.1186/1746-1340-14-10

[105] Defrin R. Chronic post-traumatic headache: clinical findings and possible mechanisms. J Man Manip Ther. 2014;22(1):36-44. doi:10.1179/2042618613Y.0000000053

Nasal Specific

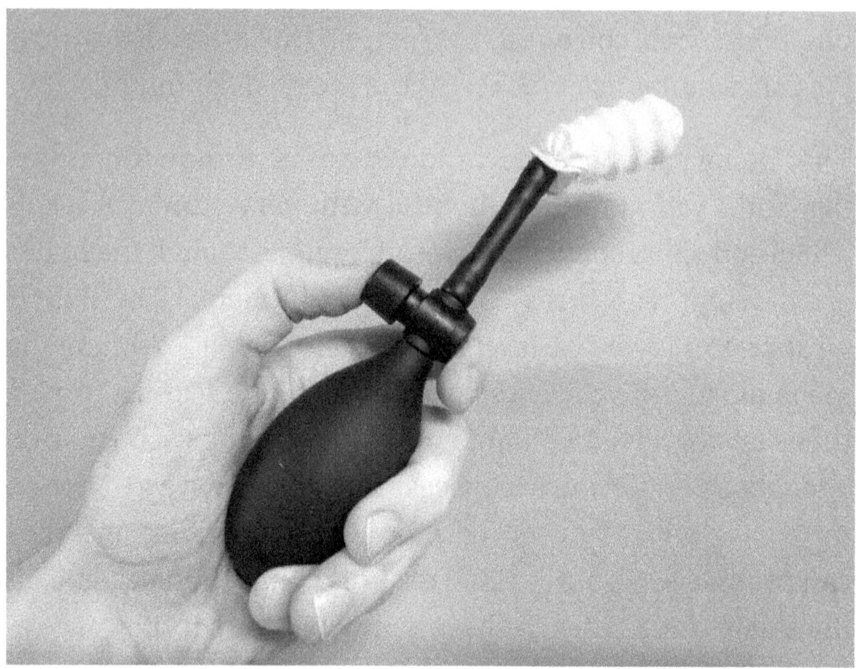

Nasal Specific can sometimes go by other names like neurocranial restructuring, etc. It involves placing a small latex balloon into the chambers of the nose. It is typically done by a naturopath, osteopath, or chiropractor although not all practitioners are trained in it. This is considered to be the ultimate cranial technique because it exerts a force underneath the sphenoid, the central cranial bone under the brain. Some claim this is an all-natural facelift and it shifts the bones of the skull.[106] Some claim it makes you better at math and improves your memory, as they allege that a more mobile sphenoid improves cerebral spinal fluid flow.[107] Like

---

[106] https://www.lsfo.co.uk/about/neurocranial-restructuring/

[107] https://www.yourhealthinmotion.com/nasal-specific-technique/

other cranial techniques, these claims are not well supported. But I've seen it help a little for those with more stubborn post-concussion and/or headache symptoms. In my experience, it almost always greatly helps with sinus issues: headaches, post-nasal drip, etc. with over an 80% success rate. Basically, unless they needed surgery to change something structural, like removing a polyp, this technique greatly reduced their symptoms. I had one person who became outraged that we didn't advertise this treatment, saying, "I've been suffering for two years! What about all the other people suffering out there that don't know about this?"

It does frustrate me that medical doctors (ENTs) don't do this. They will use a balloon during sinus surgery into the sinus cavities but they won't use a balloon into the nose cavities. Maybe it is because of the pseudoscientific explanations surrounding this technique? This technique has been around for over 80 years and is relatively safe except for those with extreme bone weakening or children (small noses and can't follow directions).

There are 6 total chambers in the nasal cavity so the lubricated latex balloon is placed into each one, one at a time, and inflated, then deflated quickly. Because of the lubricant, it feels like water going up your nose: unpleasant but not painful. All 6 chambers can be done in about 2 minutes.

Kinesio Tape

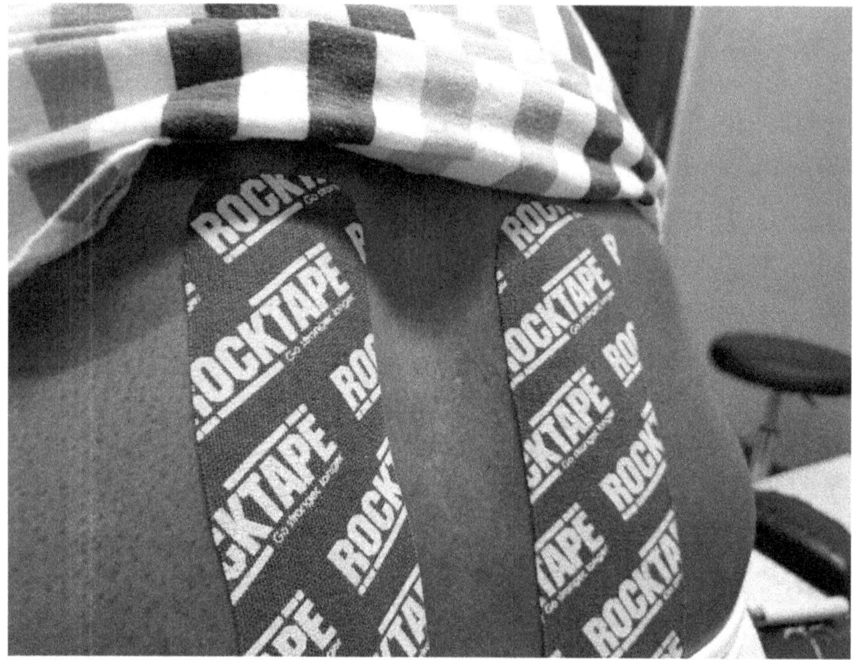

This is a stretchy tape. It does not provide the support that an athletic tape or Leukotape will. Rigid tapes or braces are recommended if you need to keep something from moving to prevent further damage, like a fresh ankle sprain. Kinesio tape is not supportive, nor rigid. It is very comfortable and normally allows for full motion of the joint, so why wear it?

This tape may reduce pain, decrease muscle tension, reduce swelling, and improve joint coordination/mobility. The evidence for any of this is of poor quality and is weak. When you add that many studies have found no benefit with using the Kinesio tape, some conclude that there is insufficient evidence to recommend it.[108] All that being said, many still use

---

[108] Parreira Pdo C, Costa Lda C, Hespanhol LC Jr, Lopes AD, Costa LO. Current evidence does not support the use of Kinesio Taping in clinical practice: a

it and it is more available now than ever. It is relatively cheap, lasts for days, and there is little risk unless you are allergic to the adhesive. I normally remove it after 3 days because I find it gets itchy. Some people notice no difference but others swear there must be some form of medication mixed into the adhesive. They won't leave until I've given them some.

There are a couple different explanations for the mechanism, but I suspect any benefit is from the pulling on the skin. The sensation of the tape can distract the nervous system from pain. The increased sensation as you stretch the tape may inform the brain more clearly where the limb is (proprioception). Improved proprioception can help decrease central sensitization (causes the brain to worry less about the area) and improves joint control. I like using it on myself for minor injuries. It doesn't get in the way, **it feels protective/supportive**, and it reminds myself that I have a minor injury, so I'm less likely to forget and do something stupid to reinjure myself.

systematic review. *J Physiother.* 2014;60(1):31-39. doi:10.1016/j.jphys.2013.12.008

Vibration Plate (Whole-Body-Vibration, WBV)

Vibration plates are platforms you stand on that vibrate. Both my mother and aunt were each conned into buying one by a door-to-door salesman. They were told that just standing on it while watching television was the same as running a marathon. I see other claims online of 10 minutes = 1 hour of cardio.[109] While the outrageous claims are false, there are some benefits to vibration plates, in particular for those with a chronic pain syndrome.[110]

If someone's pain spreads further than I expect, is more intense than it should be, or they jump in pain from a non-painful stimulus, like just touching the skin, then I throw them on the vibration plate. More often than not they like it, and when I resume my work, their body responds more normally. My personal/clinical experience is with the vertical motion plates, not the alternating vibration models which have become more plentiful and cost-effective. I typically have my patients stand normally on the vibration plate which is sufficient for whole body vibrations for a vertical vibration unit, but squatting with knees on elbows can transfer vibrations to the upper body for one of the alternating units.[111] To target shoulders, I have had people hold

---

[109] https://www.radiancestl.com/pages/faq-whole-body-vibration

[110] Wang, W., Wang, S., Lin, W. et al. Efficacy of whole body vibration therapy on pain and functional ability in people with non-specific low back pain: a systematic review. *BMC Complement Med Ther* 20, 158 (2020). https://doi.org/10.1186/s12906-020-02948-x

[111] Tsukahara Y, Iwamoto J, Iwashita K, Shinjo T, Azuma K, Matsumoto H. What is the most effective posture to conduct vibration from the lower to the

a plank on their knees before with their hands on the plate. Based on my personal and clinical experience, I would say about 12-30 Hz seems to be ideal, but you can experiment with 6-50 Hz.

Traction and Inversion Tables

Traction is the act of stretching a joint with a steady force. While this can be done for any joint, typically it refers to the neck (cervical traction) or the low back (lumbar traction). Traction is very commonly done by physiotherapists and chiropractors. About 75% of physiotherapists in the states use it, but in systematic reviews, they have not found any strong evidence supporting its use.[112,113] Clinically, I will say that it is very relieving in the short term and patients normally love it, but I have been using it less in practice and replacing it with other interventions in hopes of making my time more effective, and, if anything, my patients have been getting better faster following this change. I almost always throw it in if I have time to spare, though. I also think there is a small subset of people who respond extremely well to this therapy, and with consistent use, their pain has re-

upper extremities during whole-body vibration exercise?. *Open Access J Sports Med.* 2016;7:5-10. Published 2016 Jan 6. doi:10.2147/OAJSM.S93047

[112] Vanti C, Panizzolo A, Turone L, et al. Effectiveness of Mechanical Traction for Lumbar Radiculopathy: A Systematic Review and Meta-Analysis. *Phys Ther.* 2021;101(3):pzaa231. doi:10.1093/ptj/pzaa231

[113] Alrwaily, M., Almutiri, M. & Schneider, M. Assessment of variability in traction interventions for patients with low back pain: a systematic review. *Chiropr Man Therap* 26, 35 (2018). https://doi.org/10.1186/s12998-018-0205-z

solved and/or has not returned. When you only have a subset of people who benefit greatly, it sometimes doesn't show up in the research studies. There are some who love it, but relapse soon after the treatment is over. Their pain is worse and/or they "throw out" their neck or back soon after treatment. My theory is that the treatment relaxes the muscles, but what if the body doesn't want the muscles to be relaxed? What if those muscles were tight because the neck/back has poor segmental joint control, so the brain was protectively contracting the larger muscles for fear of injury? If those muscles don't retighten right away, maybe later that evening, the patient moves their back or neck and the coordination isn't good enough, so the muscle coordination messes up and the joint goes too far, causing more muscle spasms/pain. I now follow up traction with exercises, and this seems to prevent those relapses. I also do not perform traction anymore with severe, acute, spasming muscles (such as on the day when someone throws out their neck or back) as there is little point in my mind.

An inversion table is a way to get full spine traction along with ankles, knees, and hips. It allows you to hang upside down so gravity stretches you out. It is a fairly common at-home traction device and I cautiously recommend it to my patients. The only downside compared to other modes of traction is the blood rushing to your head may give you a headache or eye discomfort.

Hyperbaric Oxygen Therapy

Hyperbaric Oxygen Therapy (HBOT) is when you are in a chamber at elevated air pressure with increased oxygen concentration. Initially used to treat decompression sickness in divers, it surprisingly has been used and studied for chronic neuromusculoskeletal pain. It seems to have an analgesic effect.[114] In one systematic review/meta-analysis of fibromyalgia patients (central sensitization), HBOT seemed to decrease their pain, but 24% had adverse reactions.[115] They recommended looking for chambers below 2 ATM absolute air pressure which would reduce the risk of adverse events. One study looked at the effects on the brain and found that those who reported reduced pain had some changes in the regions of the brain related to fibromyalgia/central sensitization.[116]

[114] Schiavo S, DeBacker J, Djaiani C, Bhatia A, Englesakis M, Katznelson R. Mechanistic Rationale and Clinical Efficacy of Hyperbaric Oxygen Therapy in Chronic Neuropathic Pain: An Evidence-Based Narrative Review. *Pain Res Manag.* 2021;2021:8817504. doi:10.1155/2021/8817504

[115] Chen X, You J, Ma H, et al. Efficacy and safety of hyperbaric oxygen therapy for fibromyalgia: a systematic review and meta-analysis, *BMJ Open* 2023;13:e062322. doi: 10.1136/bmjopen-2022-062322

[116] Pejic W, Frey N. Hyperbaric Oxygen Therapy for the Treatment of Chronic Pain: A Review of Clinical Effectiveness and Cost-Effectiveness [Internet]. *Ottawa (ON): Canadian Agency for Drugs and Technologies in Health*; 2018 Sep 17. Available from: https://www.ncbi.nlm.nih.gov/books/NBK537956/

COMMON TYPES OF MEDICAL IMAGING

Radiographs (X-rays)

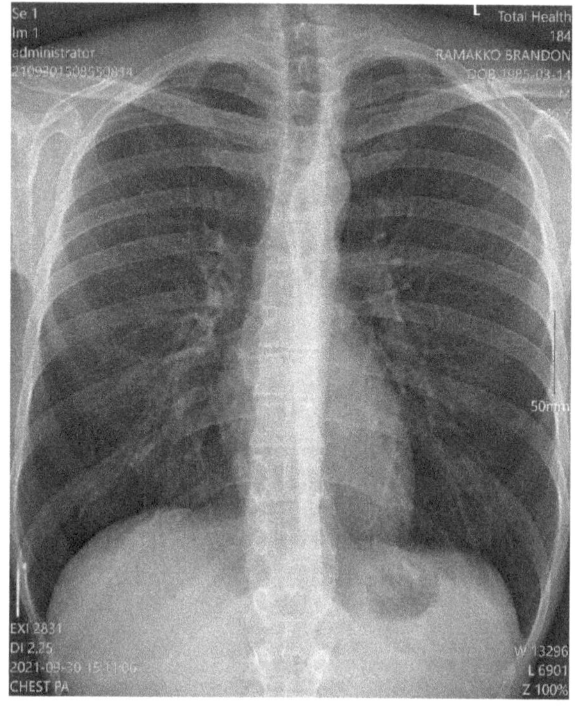

X-ray images are cheap and easy to take. X-rays are high energy photons beyond the visible spectrum. These photons of light have greater penetrating power through tissues compared to normal light that just stops at the skin. These photons have so much energy that if they do interact with your tissue, they can cause DNA damage which may lead to cancer. We are constantly exposed to DNA damaging radiation, so this additional risk is normally considered negligible. Sleeping next to someone (people are radioactive!) for a year gives you the similar radiation dose as a shoulder X-ray, which is a similar extra radiation dose you get via cosmic radiation from flying in an airplane for a couple hours.[117] While the danger is negligible, when you are playing statistics, you don't want to give people too many X-rays. When they come up with mammogram (breast X-ray scan) policies, there is always the debate about how many they catch versus how many will be caused: getting scanned daily for cancer would cause more cancers than scanning yearly, for example.

X-rays create a 2D image. The sensor records the photons that make it through the tissue. This creates a black and white image. Typically, structures are imaged in 2 planes perpendicular to each other, such as from the front and then from the side. Because you have an image of everything in the body overlapped on top of each other, it is very easy to miss a diagnosis and things in front can obfuscate things behind, and vice-versa. X-rays are used mostly for bones because they block X-rays the best, so the contrast between bone and the soft tissue is very high. You can dial in the settings so the soft tissue stuff basically disappears and you are left with only the bones. While X-rays have some limited use for some soft tissue stuff (lungs, intestines, breasts) they do not show cartilage, ligaments, tendons, or discs unless these

---

[117] Wikipedia contributors. Flight-time equivalent dose. Wikipedia, The Free Encyclopedia. August 15, 2023, 01:44 UTC. Accessed October 11, 2023. Available at: https://en.wikipedia.org/w/index.php?title=Flight-time_equivalent_dose&oldid=1170438553.

tissues have started to calcify. Normally, X-ray images can catch bone fractures and large pieces of bone missing from infection or cancer. Arthritis is often diagnosed based on X-ray. They look to see if the joint space is narrower than they expect and/or there are changes in the shape of the bone. They can't see the cartilage, though. Keep in mind that you are not a picture. I have arthritis in my neck, hands, and feet on X-ray, but I don't have constant pain in those regions.

Computed Tomography (CT or CAT scans)

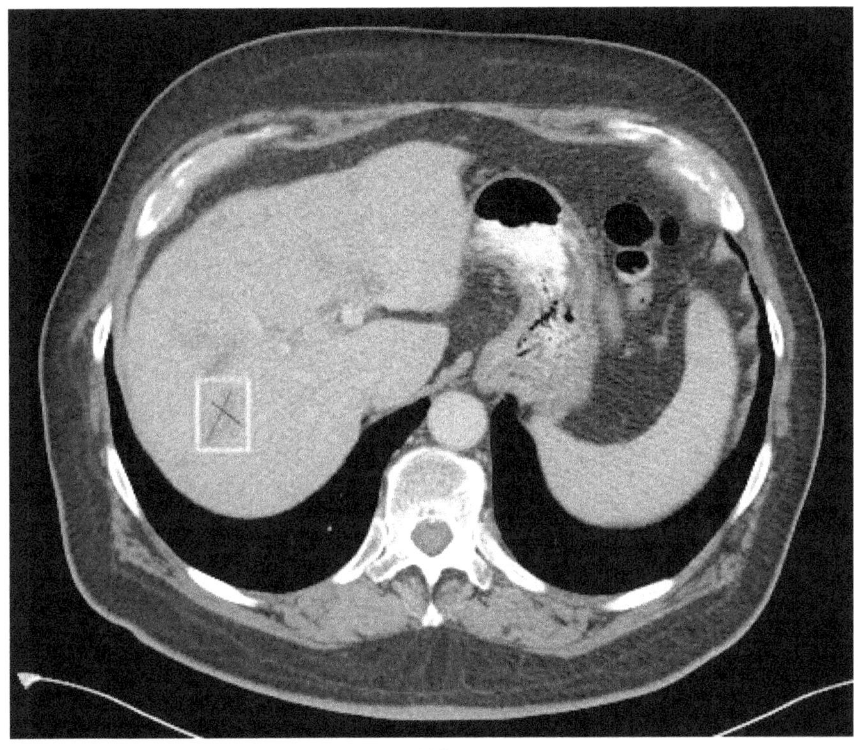

118

If you take many X-rays from different perspectives, a computer can use the information to create a 3d model of the body. A Computed Tomography (CT) scan will produce a 3D model which may be useful on its own, but slices through this model are often more useful for diagnosis. Maybe a bone has a tiny crack on the outside of it but, by looking at slices, you can follow that crack to see how far it goes. CTs are arguably the best for bones. They can be pretty good for

118 Ke Yan, Xiaosong Wang, Le Lu, Ronald M. Summers, "DeepLesion: Automated Mining of Large-Scale Lesion Annotations and Universal Lesion Detection with Deep Learning", *Journal of Medical Imaging* 5(3), 036501 (2018), doi: 10.1117/1.JMI.5.3.036501

soft tissues too, although the contrast between the tissues isn't great. They are the imaging method of choice to find brain bleeds if someone hits their head. They are relatively quick, taking a few minutes or so. The radiation dose is much higher than for a single X-ray image ($\gtrsim$10x the dose). They are better than X-rays for bones. They are better than MRI sometimes because it is cheaper and faster. CT is not very good for ligaments, tendons, and discs. CT can be more useful than MRI for moving structures like lungs and intestines where the movement would cause blurring for an MRI.

Magnetic Resonance Imaging (MRI)

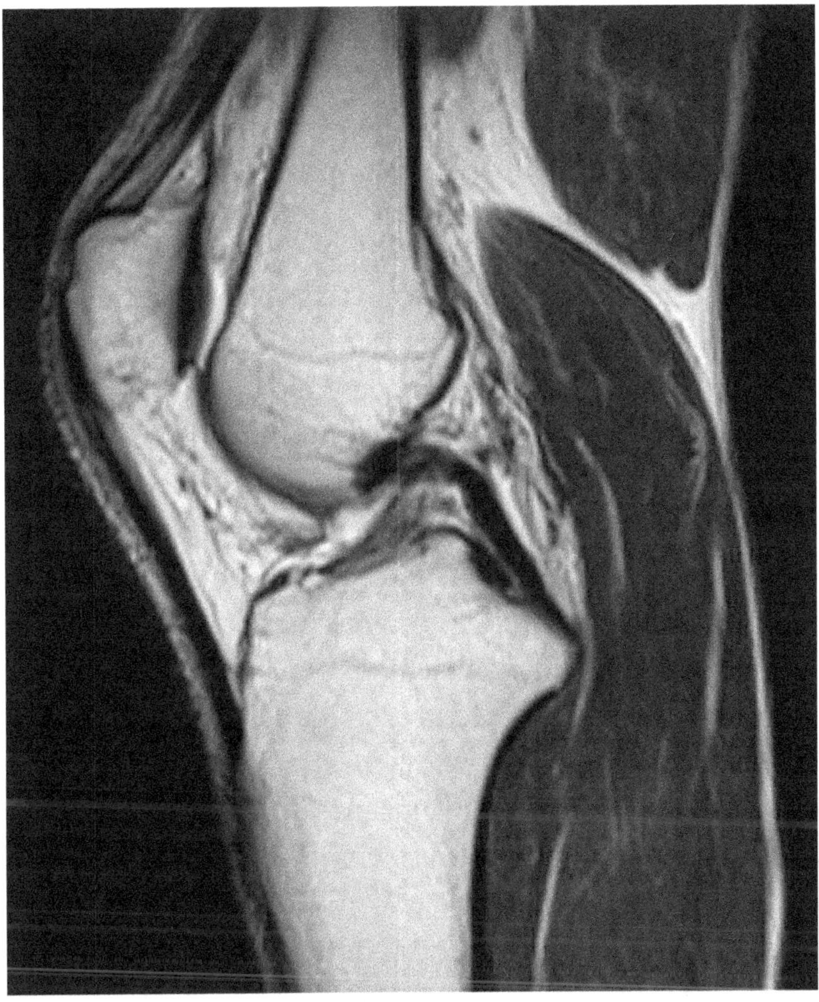

Magnetic Resonance Imaging (MRI) uses very strong magnetic fields to affect the molecules. When the molecules return to their original state, they give off a signal that the machine can interpret.[119] The magnets are typically

---

[119] This two-sentence explanation is borderline misleading due to the details left out. Even for a physicist, the exact way it works for the different types of MRI images: T1, T2, STIR, functional MRI, etc. it can get a little complicated.

electromagnets which use superconducting material that needs to be cooled with liquid helium. The machinery is loud and the images take a few minutes each to produce. If the body moves while being imaged, the image will be blurry, so your lungs breathing or your intestines pushing food through them can't be imaged well with MRI.

MRI produces slices through the body, similar to CT scan slices. It is great for seeing within tissues. Depending on the settings, the brightness of different tissues can be changed. For example, on a T1-type image, fluid is dark, and on T2-type it is bright. Taking a copy of both makes it extremely clear where the fluid is. Adding in a contrast agent can make some structures "pop" on the images. For most problems, MRIs are the best... but they are slow, and expensive, and you might have to wait a long time for an appointment depending on how many machines your city/hospital has. They only take a static picture, so if your problem involves nerves and only happens with you standing you might need to seek out a standing MRI (most are lie-down machines) so they can image the structures while you are experiencing the symptoms. MRIs are great for the discs of the spine, the spinal canal, nerve roots, and tendons. They can show tendon tears clearly (particularly if contrast is used). The contrast of the MRI is arguably better than ultrasound, but ultrasound shows most structures in greater detail and overall can be roughly equivalent for tendons and ligaments.

For some more information: Berger A. Magnetic resonance imaging. *BMJ*. 2002;324(7328):35. doi:10.1136/bmj.324.7328.35

Ultrasound Imaging (Sonography)

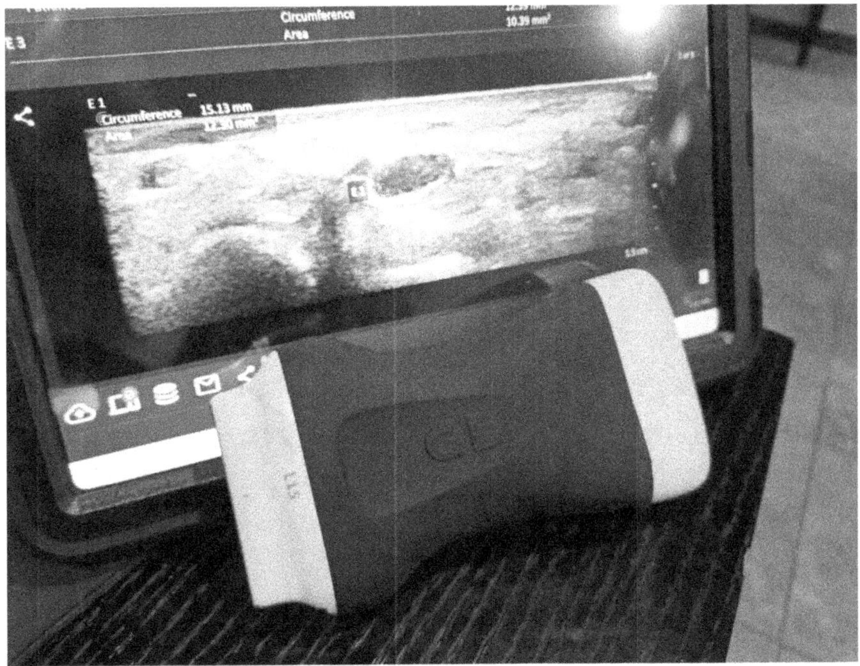

When you talk about sonography, most people think of imaging fetuses within pregnant women. As the technology has gotten better, they have developed ultrasound transducers which are very high resolution that can image the structure within a tendon or within a nerve. Imaging nerves, tendons, ligaments, and muscles is not trained within a standard sonographer program. This musculoskeletal (MSK) specialty is still in its infancy. In the states, the certification has only been around since 2012: RMSK for physician level certification and RMSKS for sonographer level certification. At its best, ultrasound imaging is better than MRI but at times useless. However, it is extremely cheap and fast. The ultrasound images a tiny slice of tissue and can't see very deep at high resolutions. The images are taken in real time and there can be benefits to imaging while the structures are moved. I can watch two parts of a torn tendon move further apart, watch something get pinched, etc. The skill of the sonographer to scan through and catch any abnormalities is key.

There are now much cheaper handheld ultrasounds. It is great that physiotherapists, chiropractors, and orthopedic surgeons are now taking quick looks inside the body with handheld ultrasound units the size of a cellphone. The quality of the image is decreased and the possibility of misdiagnosing or missing something subtle goes up, but obvious things like large tears and bad tendinosis are clearly identifiable. An image is better than no image if you understand its limitations.

Ultrasound is virtually 100% accurate at diagnosing plantar fasciosis and carpal tunnel syndrome as the plantar fascia and the median nerve both swell and noticeably darken when problematic. Ultrasound is great for muscles and tendons. It is good for hands, wrists, knees, feet, elbows, and nerves. It's okay for hips (hips can be too deep to see clearly). Unlike x-rays, ultrasound can see cartilage, which makes it arguably better for checking for arthritis. Ultrasound is roughly equivalent to MRI for shoulders and superficial structures in skilled hands.

I had a patient come in with increased hamstring pain, and he thought he strained it. He said he has had hamstring pain for years in this leg and has never been able to stretch it without pain. I scanned through and identified two regions of scar tissue, one muscle knot, and one tear. I then aggressively treated the scar tissue (x-friction) and the muscle knot (ischemic compression) while making sure not to touch the tear. If I didn't have the ultrasound image, could I have had the confidence to differentiate all four tender regions? I rescanned after treatment and everything but the tear looked approximately normal again. He actually left being able to flex his leg further than he could in a decade despite the tear, just because all the other issues were now gone.

Ultrasound is such a powerful tool. It may be worth seeking out practitioners who use it in practice. Someday ultrasounds may be as ubiquitous as the stethoscope in healthcare.

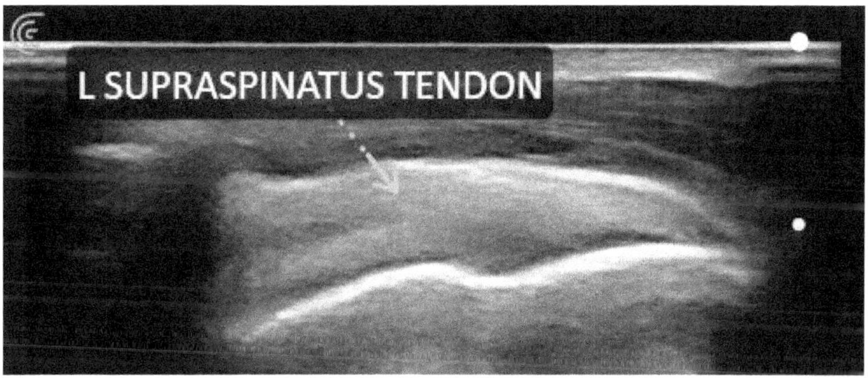

Positron Emission Tomography (PET) Scan

This is a very science fiction sounding imaging method useful for searching the whole body for things. Typically, it shows sugar/energy use, so growing cancerous tumors or infections are easily revealed. It uses a radioactive element that emits anti-matter. The anti-matter interacts with normal matter resulting in their total annihilation. The annihilated matter turns into energy (energy = mc^2) in the form of two gamma photons which must travel in opposite directions to conserve momentum. The gamma photons are then measured by a gamma camera, making the image.

Bone Scintigraphy/Scan

This is very similar to a PET scan except targeted specifically to bones. You are injected with a radioactive element that emits the gamma photons for the gamma camera. The bone scan will show areas where the bone is actively repairing. Bone tumors and fracture sites can show up clearly. This can catch bone fractures that other imaging techniques can miss.

Dual-energy X-ray Absorptiometry (DEXA) Scan

This is an X-ray scan to measure bone density, done on women as they age to gauge loss of bone strength. You get two numbers from these tests. The t-score compares you to a young healthy individual of the same sex and the z-score compares you to someone your own age and sex. Negatives are bad and positives are good. Osteoporosis is typically diagnosed when the t-score is less than -2.5.[120]

---

[120] https://www.bonehealthandosteoporosis.org/patients/diagnosis-information/bone-density-examtesting/

COMMON MEDICATIONS

The following section contains over-the-counter and prescription drugs commonly recommended to those with chronic pain. This is not an exhaustive list, nor is it an in-depth examination of each one. This section could make up half the book if I went into pharmacist-level detail. Some specific drug information is taken from Drugs.com which is a good resource for any drug. In general, you shouldn't change your prescribed medication without consulting your doctor, but in particular, some of these medications form a chemical dependence, and so coming off the medication should be done carefully/slowly. I'm not anti-drug in general. I'm anti-drug if it isn't the right drug or using drugs instead of trying to solve the problem.

Ibuprofen (Advil, Motrin, Nurofen, etc.)

This is a nonsteroidal anti-inflammatory drug (NSAID) used for pain, fever, headaches, and inflammation. This is best used only for short durations for acute injuries/pain. **Long term use can be fatal**.

"NSAIDs are not recommended for long-term use, and a careful surveillance to monitor for toxicity and efficacy is critical. Each year in the USA, the side-effects of long-term NSAID use cause nearly 103,000 hospitalizations and 16,500 deaths. This figure is similar to the annual number of deaths from AIDS and considerably greater than the number of deaths from asthma and cervical cancer."[121]

Side effects could include ulcers, gastrointestinal bleeding, high blood pressure, kidney impairment, headaches, dizziness, indigestion, heart failure/attacks, etc. Typical dose is 200-400mg every 4-6 hours. The maximum amount for adults is 800 milligrams per dose or 3200 mg per day.

Diclofenac (Voltaren gel or pills)

This is a nonsteroidal anti-inflammatory drug (NSAID) used for pain, fever, headaches, and inflammation. It has similar use and warnings to ibuprofen. It should only be used short term as it can be fatal, particularly with chronic use. It is hard on the stomach and on the heart, so it can cause internal bleeding, heart attack, or stroke.

Side effects could include headache, stomach pain, nausea, dizziness, increased blood pressure, etc. Various versions of the drug can have different usages, side effects, and recommended dosages. See the label or Drugs.com for more information.

Acetylsalicylic Acid (Aspirin)

Aspirin is another NSAID used for pain, fever, and/or inflammation. It also affects platelets, so it has anti-clotting properties. Since it has anti-clotting properties, you don't

---

[121] Ussai S, Miceli L, Pisa FE, et al. Impact of potential inappropriate NSAIDs use in chronic pain. *Drug Des Devel Ther.* 2015; 9:2073-2077. doi:10.2147/DDDT.S80686

want to take it if you have a bleeding disorder or if you are already on a blood thinner.

Side effects might include headache, upset stomach, or drowsiness. Due to its anti-clotting nature, be cautious for signs of internal bleeding: bloody stools, coughing up blood, stomach pain, etc. Dose varies wildly and may be individualized. Doses go from 50mg to 4g/day. For anti-clotting effects doses are around 80-160mg and for pain 325-650mg every 4-6 hours with a max of 4g/day.

Celecoxib (Celebrex)

This is a nonsteroidal anti-inflammatory drug (NSAID) used for pain, tenderness, swelling, and stiffness. In particular, this is the go-to drug for arthritis related symptoms. Unlike the other NSAIDs on my list, this NSAID is in a different category (Cox-2 inhibitor). It does not have the awful, and potentially lethal, gastrointestinal side effects that other NSAIDs have.

Related drugs have been associated with increased chances of heart attack, but celecoxib is considered safe at the recommended dosages. There are mild and varied side effects, but the most common are dizziness and constipation. Typical dose is 100-400mg. For arthritis, 200mg/day is normally prescribed.

In my 20s I was prescribed Celecoxib/Celebrex in perpetuity for joint pain and inflammation in my hands, knees, and feet. This is a very strong and effective drug: night-and-day difference between this and Advil. It allowed me to start being active again. It allowed me to be able to walk mostly pain free again. The only side effect was when I first took it, I had trouble sleeping that night (very rare side effect). Still... I didn't like the idea of being on drugs my whole life. By experimenting with my diet and by doing some rehab exercises for my knees, I was able to be pain free without the drugs.

Acetaminophen (Tylenol, paracetamol, Anacin, Excedrin, etc.)

This is a pain and fever reducer. It is a very common pain reliever that is the active pain-relieving ingredient in many combination medications like Robaxacet. An overdose can damage the liver or cause death. A recommended dose of Tylenol (2 extra strength capsules) is 1000mg/6 hours, which is the maximum dose! Do not exceed this! If you are a petite woman, use less. It should not be taken with alcohol.

Initial signs of overdose could be loss of appetite, nausea, vomiting, stomach pain, sweating, and confusion/weakness. Later symptoms might be pain in your upper stomach, dark urine, and yellowing of your skin (jaundice). A typical dose is roughly 500-1000mg every 6 hours. The maximum for adults is 1000mg/dose and 4000mg/day.

Opioids (Tramadol, Oxycodone, Codeine, hydrocodone, morphine, etc.)

Opioids are addictive. They should be prescribed carefully and their use should be minimized. They are extremely effective pain relievers, though. There are potentially lethal complications with taking these with alcohol or sedatives: they can stop your breathing. They are prescribed as needed or in extended-release versions which are taken once a day. Tylenol-3 is Tylenol mixed with codeine.

The most common side effects are drowsiness, constipation, nausea, dizziness, tiredness, etc. Dosage varies wildly depending on the type of opioid and most doctors start the patient as low as possible.

Benzodiazepines (diazepam/Valium, alprazolam/Xanax, etc.)

These drugs are addictive. They are used to treat anxiety disorders, insomnia, or alcohol withdrawal symptoms. They are sometimes used to treat muscle spasms/stiffness or seizures. Similar to opioids, they can negatively affect breathing. These work via neurotransmitters and can have neurological side effects such as panic attacks, confusion, paranoia, seizures, insomnia, irritability, aggressiveness, talkativeness, or suicidal thoughts. Withdrawal symptoms can last as long as 12 months.

Common, more benign effects are drowsiness and muscle weakness. The typical dosage of diazepam for muscle spasms or anxiety is 2-10mg, 2-4 times/day.

Muscle Relaxers (Baclofen, Carisoprodol, Cyclobenzaprine, Methocarbamol/Robaxin, etc.)

The action of all these drugs is similar to that of benzos (diazepam/Valium). Whereas diazepam is normally prescribed for anxiety with a side effect of muscle weakness, muscle relaxers are prescribed primarily for the muscle anti spasm effects. Muscle relaxers are GABA agonists. They help GABA inhibit signaling. So, the signaling in the body is depressed. This can have mental effects (drowsiness), intestinal effects (constipation), and the intended effect of weaker/looser muscles. They slow everything down. Most muscle relaxers are for short term use only and are limited to 2-3 weeks.

I'm not a fan of muscle relaxers. This opinion comes from personal experience and patient reports. When my neck would lock up and pain was 10/10 when I tried to move, the muscle relaxers didn't seem to help. When I ask most patients if they feel the drugs are helping, more often than not say no. I find that even if they do work, some people can't tolerate the side effects. If your muscles are chronically tight and protective, it is better to work on why instead of the Band-aid solution.

Gabapentin

Gabapentin has only been approved for post-herpetic nerve pain from shingles, seizures, and restless leg syndrome. Gabapentin is very, very commonly prescribed, off-label, for nerve pain. Off-label means it hasn't been approved for that use by the FDA. For the population of patients I see in my clinic, maybe 20% of people who come in telling me they have nerve pain actually have nerve pain (muscle-referred pain can mimic nerve pain pretty convincingly). A recent study found that those who visited a chiropractor for back pain were about 50% less likely to receive an off-label gabapentin prescription.[122] My own experience and this study make me question how over prescribed this drug might be. Most fibromyalgia patients I've worked with have been on Gabapentin and a subset have told me it had helped them.

The mechanism of gabapentin is similar to benzos and muscle relaxers so the side effects and risks are similar. Common side effects are chills, sore throat, body aches, tiredness, headache, swelling in the legs, trouble speaking, vision problems, dizziness, drowsiness, tremors, unsteadiness, nausea, etc.

Antidepressants/SSRIs (Lexapro, Zoloft, Prozac, Paxil, Sarafem, etc.)

Selective Serotonin Reuptake Inhibitors (SSRIs) are a class of antidepressants and often the go-to prescription for depression. They are sometimes prescribed to those with a chronic pain disorder/fibromyalgia as well. These drugs do

---

[122] Trager RJ, Cupler ZA, Srinivasan R, Casselberry RM, Perez JA, Dusek JA. Association between chiropractic spinal manipulation and gabapentin prescription in adults with radicular low back pain: retrospective cohort study using US data. *BMJ Open*. 2023;13(7):e073258. Published 2023 Jul 21. doi:10.1136/bmjopen-2023-073258

cause some chemical dependence, so coming off the drug too quickly can cause depression or manic episodes. Rare side effects are severe depression and suicide. The body likes to maintain a certain balance of hormones, and when a drug tries to make changes, the body adapts by changing the amount produced or the number of receptors. This is why it is hard to stop antidepressants because the body has to undo the modifications it made while on the drug.

SSRIs are not more effective than placebo for the majority of patients.[123] They are only more effective in the most severe cases of depression, and even then, it was statistically significant, but not clinically significant.[124] But doctors can't prescribe placebos. So, what is the doctor supposed to do, not prescribe a drug? That's crazy talk! (For the record, placebos and SSRIs both helped, and if you have had success and are on them, do not stop suddenly as it is dangerous to do so. Talk to your doctor.)

I encourage people to try other things first if they are considering prescription antidepressants, particularly for mild

---

[123] Mayor S. Meta-analysis shows difference between antidepressants and placebo is only significant in severe depression. *BMJ*. 2008;336(7642):466. doi:10.1136/bmj.39503.656852.DB

[124] Jakobsen J, et al. . Selective serotonin reuptake inhibitors versus placebo in patients with major depressive disorder. A systematic review with meta-analysis and Trial Sequential Analysis. *BMC Psychiatry*. 17. (2017) 10.1186/s12888-016-1173-2.

to moderate depression. **Mental health therapy**[125] or **exercise**[126] both work as well as antidepressants. **St. John's Wort** (botanical remedy) **works as well as antidepressants for major depressive disorders, and with fewer side effects.**[127]

Proton-pump Inhibitors (Prilosec/omeprazole and other prazoles)

Proton-pump inhibitors work by preventing the release of acid ions into your stomach. This class of drugs might seem an odd choice to include in this list, but my pharmacology instructor was on a crusade against misuse of these drugs, and I seem to have been converted to her cause. They are recommended for short term use but many individuals are prescribed them forever, which can lead to health repercussions. If the problem is an ulcer, they are usually prescribed correctly, where they are taken until it is healed. That isn't the case for acid reflux. Acid reflux, also called gastroesophageal reflux disease (GERD), is when the sphincter (muscle

[125] Cuijpers, P., Noma, H., Karyotaki, E., Vinkers, C.H., Cipriani, and Furukawa, T.A. A network meta-analysis of the effects of psychotherapies, pharmacotherapies and their combination in the treatment of adult depression. *World Psychiatry,* (2020) 19: 92-107. https://doi.org/10.1002/wps.20701

[126] Recchia F, Leung CK, Chin EC, *et al.* Comparative effectiveness of exercise, antidepressants and their combination in treating non-severe depression: a systematic review and network meta-analysis of randomized controlled trials. *British Journal of Sports Medicine* 2022; 56:1375-1380.

[127] Apaydin, E.A., Maher, A.R., Shanman, R. et al. A systematic review of St. John's wort for major depressive disorder. *Syst Rev* 5, 148 (2016). https://doi.org/10.1186/s13643-016-0325-2

controlling the opening and closing at the top of the stomach) isn't keeping the contents of your stomach from coming back up the esophagus. This leads to stomach acid burning and eroding the lining of the esophagus. Over time, this can damage the nerves controlling the sphincter, making the problem worse. Ultimately, this can lead to cancer of the esophagus. So, there is a reason doctors prescribe this drug, considering how severe the problem can get. What is supposed to happen is they are supposed to use proton-pump inhibitors for short term symptom relief while they advise the patient on lifestyle modifications. The proton pump inhibitor doesn't stop the reflux, it just makes it less painful and less damaging. Advice like eating smaller meals (the stomach is smaller than you think), not lying down within 30 minutes of eating, modifying diet, etc. might be all it takes to eliminate this problem at its source.

Common side effects of these drugs are cold-type symptoms, stomach pain, gas, nausea, diarrhea, and headache. Typically, you will have less than half the available acid for food digestion, so with chronic use you will develop nutrient deficiencies because you are not digesting your food properly. You may develop osteoporosis (bone weakening), a magnesium deficiency (dizziness, muscle spasms, irregular heartbeat, etc.), vitamin B-12 deficiency (muscle weakness, fatigue, pins and needles, etc.), and more. It is also tough on the kidneys.

Statins (Lipitor, Altoprev, pravastatin, Crestor, etc.)

Statins are a class of drugs for reducing cholesterol levels in the blood prescribed to those with a high risk of having cardiovascular events. Statins do save lives, but they should be a second line of defense. Lifestyle modifications (diet and increased activity) are superior to statins and come with other beneficial effects.[128]

Statins increase the risk of developing diabetes. Common side effects of statins are headache, excessive gas, constipation, indigestion, nausea, lower back or flank pain, muscle pain/tenderness, weakness, face pain/tenderness, stuffy nose, sweating, insomnia, difficulty with urination, etc.

---

[128] Becker DJ, French B, Morris PB, Silvent E, Gordon RY. Phytosterols, red yeast rice, and lifestyle changes instead of statins: a randomized, double-blinded, placebo-controlled trial. *Am Heart J.* 2013;166(1):187-196. doi:10.1016/j.ahj.2013.03.019

COMMON BOTANICALS AND NATURAL REMEDIES

The following section contains common supplements and botanicals recommended to those with chronic pain. This is not an exhaustive list, nor is it an in-depth examination of each one. Unless otherwise noted, information is taken from Healthnotes. In general, supplements and botanicals rarely have any good-quality research done on them. Avoid homeopathic concoctions unless you want a placebo.

St. John's Wort

This is an herb found in Europe and western North America; this herb seems to be equivalent to medical antidepressants with fewer side effects. The exact mechanism is debated and there may be overlapping mechanisms at play. For mild to moderate **depression,** 500-1200mg is recommended. It may take 2 weeks to start taking effect. One study found it helpful for **anxiety** as well. A St. John's Wort cream can be helpful for **eczema**.

Glucosamine/Chondroitin Sulphate

Both of these supplements are building blocks of cartilage. They both seem to slow the progression of cartilage degradation (osteoarthritis). In most studies (not all) they improved pain and function in those diagnosed with **osteoarthritis**.[129,130] The resulting symptom relief can take months and continued use may be required. Luckily the body tolerates these supplements very well. Chondroitin also may lower blood cholesterol levels as an added bonus. I personally took these for 3 months and didn't notice a difference in my joint pain. For me, changing my diet and taking a few other supplements on this list did eliminate my joint pain. One theme in this book is that you might have to try multiple solutions to find one that works for you. For osteoarthritis, the typical dose of chondroitin is 800-1200mg/day and 1500mg/day for glucosamine.

Curcumin (turmeric)

Turmeric is a common ingredient in Indian Curries. Curcumin is the active ingredient in turmeric. It is a potent **antioxidant** and **anti-inflammatory**. I recommend curcumin above ibuprofen and other similar NSAIDs. Curcumin has similar benefits to pain and function without the troublesome, and sometimes lethal, gastrointestinal side effects of

---

[129] Jerosch J. Effects of Glucosamine and Chondroitin Sulfate on Cartilage Metabolism in OA: Outlook on Other Nutrient Partners Especially Omega-3 Fatty Acids. *Int J Rheumatol.* 2011;2011:969012. doi:10.1155/2011/969012

[130] Čeh T, Šarabon N. Effects of adding glucosamine or glucosamine combined with chondroitin to exercise on pain and physical function in adults with knee osteoarthritis: a systematic review and meta-analysis. *Eur J Transl Myol.* 2023 Nov 23;33(4):12013. doi: 10.4081/ejtm.2023.12013

NSAIDs.[131] Curcumin isn't absorbed easily by the body, so you may find it sometimes bio-optimized in trademarked formulations or combined with piperine (black pepper) to increase its efficiency.

Comfrey

This is a traditional topical ointment made from the root of this plant. It is an effective **topical anti-inflammatory**. It is as effective as diclofenac as long as you aren't using a homeopathic version. While the tea has some traditional uses, internal ingestion of comfrey products should be avoided as the roots and young leaves are toxic to the liver.

Bromelain

This is an enzyme found in pineapples. This enzyme breaks things down. It seems to help with inflammatory conditions and injuries like sinusitis, sprains/strains, etc. You want to get the enteric coated pills taken and take them on an empty stomach or else the enzymes will get used up digesting your food instead of being absorbed into your body. There is no good evidence that there is any benefit for chronic problems.

---

[131] Paultre K, Cade W, Hernandez D, *et al.* Therapeutic effects of turmeric or curcumin extract on pain and function for individuals with knee osteoarthritis: a systematic review. *BMJ Open Sport & Exercise Medicine* 2021;7:e000935. doi: 10.1136/bmjsem-2020-000935

Cranberry Extract

Cranberry juice has been on-and-off recommended for **urinary tract infections** (UTIs). Some studies show some benefits and others don't. The issue is that cranberries contain a chemical which keeps the bacteria from sticking to the walls of the urinary tract, but sugar is bad for UTIs. In theory, taking cranberry extract would be superior to cranberry juice because it has all the benefits and none of the drawbacks. From preliminary studies and personal anecdotes from women I've recommended this to, it can prevent chronic UTIs taken regularly or in temporal proximity to intercourse.[132] It might help with active UTIs.[133]

Garlic

The predominant active medicinal component obtained from garlic is allicin. This chemical is an antioxidant and seems to help with **high blood pressure** and atherosclerosis (helps prevent heart attacks and strokes). Although not solely attributed to allicin, garlic seems to be a mild anticoagulant as well (blood thinner). Garlic doesn't actually contain allicin. It is produced by an enzyme that is released

---

[132] Babar A, Moore L, Leblanc V, et al. High dose versus low dose standardized cranberry proanthocyanidin extract for the prevention of recurrent urinary tract infection in healthy women: a double-blind randomized controlled trial. *BMC Urol.* 2021;21(1):44. Published 2021 Mar 23. doi:10.1186/s12894-021-00811-w

[133] Gbinigie OA, Spencer EA, Heneghan CJ, Lee JJ, Butler CC. Cranberry Extract for Symptoms of Acute, Uncomplicated Urinary Tract Infection: A Systematic Review. *Antibiotics (Basel).* 2020;10(1):12. Published 2020 Dec 25. doi:10.3390/antibiotics10010012

when the garlic is crushed/cut. If cooking, prepare the garlic and let it sit for 10 minutes before exposing it to heat because heat will destroy the enzyme. In one study, using 12 weeks of supplementation, they found that one third had significant reduction in blood pressure with an average drop of 11.2mmHg systolic and 6.4mmHg diastolic in the subgroup.[134] The recommended dose is typically 600-1200mg/day garlic extract. For comparison, decreasing salt intake reduces blood pressure by an average of 3.4 mmHg systolic and 1.5 mmHg diastolic.[135]

Ginger

Ginger seems to help with **nausea** from migraines, morning sickness, vertigo, motion sickness, etc. Ginger may be a mild anticoagulant (helps for blood clots) but not all research supports this. It may help with **arthritis** as, in two studies, pain was reduced compared with placebo at doses of roughly 500mg/day.

Coenzyme Q10 (CoQ10)

This enzyme is also called ubiquinone because it is ubiquitous and found throughout the body. It helps with the creation of ATP which is the unit of energy for the body. So, the

---

[134] Ried K, Travica N, Sali A. The effect of aged garlic extract on blood pressure and other cardiovascular risk factors in uncontrolled hypertensives: the AGE at Heart trial. *Integr Blood Press Control* 2016;9:9–21. doi:10.2147/IBPC.S93335

[135] Aburto NJ, Ziolkovska A, Hooper L, Elliott P, Cappuccio FP, Meerpohl JJ. Effect of lower sodium intake on health: systematic review and meta-analyses. *BMJ*. 2013;346:f1326. Published 2013 Apr 3. doi:10.1136/bmj.f1326

more CoQ10, the easier and faster the body can make ATP (provided the body has the other necessities). Supplementing with extra CoQ10 can help with **angina** (heart pain), **fibromyalgia**, and **migraines**.

Fibromyalgia is a full body chronic pain syndrome. The nervous system works overtime ramping up all that pain such that the body and nervous system is fatigued at a cellular level. Understandably fibromyalgia patients had lower levels of CoQ10. Supplementation seemed to help with the associated fatigue, pain, and headaches. In a couple of trials of migraine patients, headache frequency decreased by over 50% in roughly half the participants. The recommended dose is 150-300mg/day.

Ginseng

There are two types of ginsengs (American and Asian). While they may have similar effects, the research into ginseng is limited (especially for American ginseng) and its exact dosage/efficacy is poorly established. Ginseng may help with libido, improve athletic performance, prevent colds/flu (it is the active ingredient in COLD-FX), and may help those suffering from stress and/or a chronic fatigue syndrome. It seems to help modulate the immune system and hormones of the body improving overall function.

COMMON NUTRITIONAL SUPPLEMENTS

In general, supplements are **only beneficial if you are deficient**. Taking extra, above what you need, rarely has any harmful effects: only some could be harmful, and of those, you would need to take multiple concurrent doses to hit dangerous values. These are also things found in food so diet changes can help. Unless otherwise stated, information comes from Healthnotes.

Omega-3

Our body contains many enzymes for breaking things down into constituent parts and to build all the complicated molecules our body needs. We need enough of the base constituents or else our body will be unable to function properly. These foundational building blocks are called the essential fatty acids and the essential amino acids (In addition to essential vitamins and minerals). There are 3 of these essential fatty acids: ALA, DHA, and EPA. Technically DHA/EPA can be made from ALA but the process is not very efficient so it may be best to get DHA/EPA on its own.

There is a ton of relatively low-quality research on Omega-3 supplementation (fish oil). These fats have many uses in the body, so supplementation may have various effects. Of particular interest is the fact that the chemical messenger the body uses to control inflammation is made from them. If you don't have enough Omega-3s, then **inflammation** can run wild. Supplementation may reduce inflammation, prevent heart failure, lower triglycerides, lower blood pressure, and may help with lupus symptoms, rheumatoid arthritis, angina (heart pain), anxiety, asthma, atherosclerosis, depression, headaches, Crohn's disease, dysmenorrhea, eczema, epilepsy, multiple sclerosis (MS), obesity, osteoporosis, psoriasis, Raynaud's disease, Schizophrenia, tooth decay, etc.

How much do you need, what is ideal, what are the recommended supplement amounts? There isn't a clear answer. We probably get enough ALA in our diets; it is the other two we may need to supplement. Total values around 1.1-1.6g/daily seems to be normal/adequate, but there isn't a recommended daily value and no recommended minimum for the DHA/EPA component.[136] Most research is preliminary. They want to make sure that if there is an effect that they see it so most research goes a little overkill: 3g of DHA/EPA. This is equivalent to 10 grams of fish oil, which is a lot. Most who consume this much measure by the teaspoon instead of taking the 10 capsules. I normally recommend 2 capsules a day for everyone and 4-6 capsules a day if I think they might be deficient. Taking it with other vitamins is useful since some vitamins are fat soluble and the fat helps you absorb them.

---

[136] https://ods.od.nih.gov/factsheets/Omega3FattyAcids-HealthProfessional/

Good dietary sources of DHA/EPA are: seafood, flax seeds, chia seeds, and walnuts.[137]

Boron

Boron is an element found in trace amounts in the human body. It doesn't seem to be widely accepted as "essential" yet, but my interpretation of the research makes a strong case for its need. There is a growing amount of evidence suggesting our diets are deficient in boron which is why supplementing with boron seems to have such beneficial effects: in particular for **arthritis** and **reduced male libido**.[138] The higher quality multivitamin companies are now including boron in their multivitamins. Supplementation seems to be anywhere from 1-12mg, but I normally recommend 3-6mg. A fairly recent systematic review in 2019 concluded the following:

> "Boron has a positive effect on the growth of bone and central nervous system, hormone regulation, reducing the risk of some types of cancer, improvement of arthritis and associated heart disease symptoms, speeding up the wound healing, pain reduction in gynecological diseases, and kidney stones. Despite the need for boron intake of 1-3 mg per day in adults, symptoms of boron deficiency such as arthritis, amnesia, osteoporosis, degenerative and soft cartilage diseases, hormonal disorders, and decreased libido

---

[137] https://www.healthline.com/nutrition/12-omega-3-rich-foods

[138] Pizzorno L. Nothing Boring About Boron. *Integr Med (Encinitas)*. 2015;14(4):35-48.

are still common, and this deficiency can have many adverse effects that can be prevented. Therefore, its consumption as a reasonable dietary and a suitable alternative for common chemical drugs is recommended."[139]

Good dietary sources of boron are: prune juice, avocado, raisins, peaches, apples, pears, peanuts, beans, and grapes.[140]

Vitamin D

This vitamin's main role is managing calcium in the body. It can help the body absorb more calcium and reduces how much is excreted. Vitamin D has other roles in the body that aren't as well understood. It seems to be necessary for **proper immune-system functioning** because those deficient in vitamin D end up getting more colds, more eczema, more autoimmune conditions like MS, etc.[141] It may have an **effect on the nervous system** too, as those deficient had more fibromyalgia pain, more back pain, more epileptic seizures, worse headaches, worse mood, etc. Obese individuals typically have lower levels of vitamin D, and supplementation seemed to help with weight loss. Vitamin D seems to

---

[139] Nikkhah S, Naghii M R. Medicinal Properties of Boron Supplementation on the Prevention and Treatment of Diseases: A Systematic Review. *cmja* 2019; 9 (3) :3760-3779

[140] https://ods.od.nih.gov/factsheets/Boron-HealthProfessional/

[141] Sintzel MB, Rametta M, Reder AT. Vitamin D and Multiple Sclerosis: A Comprehensive Review. *Neurol Ther.* 2018;7(1):59-85. doi:10.1007/s40120-017-0086-4

help with pancreatic function as supplementation can help with diabetes symptoms.

This for me was one of the key supplements that helped me become pain free. I noticed a difference in the first week. Dosage may be as high as 7,000IU daily (50,000IU weekly) for a severe, established deficiency but only for 1-3 months to get you back up to normal levels. For maintenance, 1,000-4,000 IU daily is recommended. It is fat soluble, so take it with oil/food. It is often found in an oil capsule instead of a pill.

Good dietary sources of vitamin D are: cod liver oil, salmon, tuna, beef liver, eggs, and fortified food (drinks and cereals).[142] Some vitamin D can be made by this skin when exposed to UVB light. So, exposure to sunlight can help, but keep in mind UVB causes skin cancer.

Magnesium

This is an essential mineral for the body. A deficiency has been linked to cardiac arrhythmia, higher blood pressure, more frequent and intense migraines, worse nerve symptoms, asthma, ADHD, chronic fatigue, osteoporosis, muscle cramps, etc.

Just because supplementation may help muscle cramps for those who are deficient doesn't mean taking extra will help with the tight protective muscle spasms associated with the

---

[142] https://ods.od.nih.gov/factsheets/VitaminD-HealthProfessional/ , https://www.hsph.harvard.edu/nutritionsource/vitamin-d/

chronic pain and functional instability (poor muscle coordination) discussed at length in this book.

Magnesium is one of the minerals that cheap multivitamins often use an inferior version of. Magnesium oxide isn't absorbed easily but magnesium citrate, chloride, malate, lactate, L-threonate, taurate, orotate, or glycinate are all absorbed well.[143] Topical magnesium creams seem to have no effect on magnesium levels. Supplementation ranges from 200-600mg. The recommended daily amount (RDA) is 320mg for women and 420mg for men.

Good dietary sources of magnesium are: pumpkin seeds, chia seeds, almonds, cashews, peanuts, kidney/black beans, spinach, potatoes w/skin, and brown rice.[144]

B12/Folate

Vitamin B12 (methocobalamin) deficiency is most often associated with anemia. When identified, B12+folic acid+iron are typically recommended. B12 deficiency and folic acid deficiency often present the same which is why supplementation typically includes both. Some functions of B12 involve folic acid and B6.

In terms of chronic problems, a deficiency can cause **fatigue**, depression, migraines, and **nerve symptoms** (tingling, numbness, weakness). I've had half a dozen patients with bilateral nerve symptoms which improved initially via

---

[143] https://www.healthline.com/nutrition/magnesium-types

[144] https://ods.od.nih.gov/factsheets/Magnesium-HealthProfessional/

my work but then plateaued. They only resolved with B12 supplementation. A B12 deficiency is linked to decreased sperm counts, cognitive decline, and macular degeneration (vision loss).

When a deficiency is identified, typically injections are administered to get the numbers up quickly. Supplementation is rarely without the other B vitamins, folate, and/or iron. The RDA for B12 is 0.0024mg/day but supplements are often 0.003-3mg/day, typically around 1mg/day. Taking extra B vitamins is not harmful as you just urinate the extras out (urine turns bright yellow).

Good dietary sources of B12 vitamins are all animal products, so **vegans/vegetarians are normally deficient unless they supplement or consume cereals/milks/drinks fortified with B12**.[145]

Iron

Iron deficiency causes anemia which causes fatigue and worsens depression, athletic performance, and ADHD. Iron is typically no longer included in multivitamins. Supplementation is not commonly recommended as increased research suggests that regular supplementation is rarely required. Supplementation is typically only done after anemia is identified via blood test and under physician supervision.

---

[145] https://ods.od.nih.gov/factsheets/VitaminB12-HealthProfessional/ , https://www.healthline.com/nutrition/vitamin-b12-foods

Iron supplements at the supermarket more commonly take the form of energy tonics containing iron and the B vitamins/folate. Iron supplements can cause constipation and stomach cramps. Ferrous sulphate is the best version. The RDA for iron is 8mg/day but 100mg/day is often recommended in cases of deficiency until resolved.

Good dietary sources of iron are: red meat, beans, nuts, dried fruit, and liver.[146]

Zinc

Zinc is an essential mineral **necessary for injury repair**. A deficiency can greatly decrease your body's ability to heal tendons and ligaments. Zinc deficiency is also linked to an impaired immune system and male infertility. Interestingly, zinc seems to directly interfere with viruses so it is included in some cold lozenges (13-25mg as zinc gluconate, glycine, or acetate every 2 hours). Zinc RDA is 8mg/day for women and 11mg/day for men. When supplementing with zinc, copper is often also recommended, taken separately, to prevent a copper deficiency (zinc affects copper, iron, and phosphorus absorption). Signs of copper deficiency are fatigue, weakness, brittle bones, cold sensitivity, etc.

Good dietary sources of zinc are: seafood (oysters in particular), meat, legumes, milk products, and pumpkin seeds.[147]

---

[146] https://www.nhs.uk/conditions/vitamins-and-minerals/iron/

[147] https://ods.od.nih.gov/factsheets/Zinc-HealthProfessional/

Multivitamins

I typically recommend a multivitamin to most individuals. If you have a deficiency, even a cheap multivitamin might help but the more expensive multivitamins out there are better as they are more complete, may have more absorbable versions of components (like for magnesium), and may contain extra good stuff (like CoQ10). If you are doing well financially, splurge on a better one if you can. You may need to supplement in addition to the multivitamin for things like vitamin D, magnesium, Omega-3, boron, iron, etc. Plant-based diets have great benefits and are more nutritious, but even vegetarians may need supplementation like for vitamin B12. For someone who eats healthily, normally I recommend individual supplements instead of a multivitamin (B and D vitamins and omega-3s).

DECENT SOURCES OF INFORMATION

Website	Description
DrRamakko.com	This is my personal website. I have some videos and articles there. You can also book virtual sessions with me so I can answer your questions or to receive health coaching.
triggerpoints.net	You can look up where nasty muscle knots might be hiding. The website contains common muscle knot locations and their referred pain pattern. You can search by muscle or by where the pain is.
Drugs.com	A useful resource for any drugs you may be taking. Has dosage and common side effects. Has information on signs for when to call your doctor or go to emergency. Good to read through for every drug you take.
Healthnotes	A useful resource for supplement and botanical information. There is a star rating system based on how strong the evidence is. Has information on the mechanism, evidence, dosage, interactions, and side effects. https://www.nutriadvanced.co.uk/healthnotes/
Mayo clinic, Cleveland clinic, etc.	Some hospitals or clinics create resources and handouts for patients. The Mayo Clinic and Cleveland Clinic both have reasonably good basic level information on their respective websites. If I Google a diagnosis and one of their sites comes up, I often email that link to a patient.
NHS	The NHS is the UK health system and the individual hospitals create handouts for patients. I Google: "(name of health condition) NHS handout" and I nor-

	mally have a selection of handouts appropriate to provide to patients with home care advice and/or exercises.
Bob & Brad	There is lots of great stuff on YouTube, and I chose this channel as an example. This channel is a couple of physiotherapists sharing exercises and stretches that have helped their patients. Notice their use of language, "I find this helps some of my patients" or "Sometimes I have my patient do this," etc. Not every exercise is perfect for everyone or for every condition.
Physiopedia	This is a resource for physiotherapists but anyone can Google "condition+physiopedia" to find their article on how to diagnose and treat the condition. I find myself using it semi-regularly.
UWS CSPE Protocols and Care Pathways	These are the University of Western States' clinical standards, protocols, and educational resources. These are detailed documents based on the best evidence available. They describe how to diagnose and treat various conditions. Similar to Physiopedia in that it is written for health professionals. https://www.uws.edu/cspe-protocols-care-pathways/
Harvard's Nutrition Source	This is a research based nutritional resource written for the general public.
NIH Office of Dietary Supplements	This is a research based nutritional resource for both the general public and for health professionals.

PART 3:
REGION BY REGION

HEADACHES

There are over 200 types/variations of headaches as categorized by the International Headache Society, and these headaches have overlapping symptoms and the presentations can vary between patients.[148] Thankfully, most primary headaches are one of two types: Tension-type headaches and migraines. Primary refers to the fact that the pain, ultimately, comes from the brain/brainstem. After covering those, I'll briefly discuss post-concussive headaches, and then three types of secondary headaches where pain is coming from nearby structures.

The focus will be on chronic headaches, but it is important to mention that the sudden onset of a new type of headache or a progressively worsening headache associated with seizures, difficulty speaking, difficulty swallowing, difficulty with facial expression, etc. are both serious causes for concern. The former may be a sign of a brain bleed. It is often called a thunderclap headache due to their sudden arrival and extreme severity, often being described as the worst headache they've ever had. The latter can be a sign of a brain tumor. Get help if this happens to you or a loved one. Seek emergency help if signs of a brain bleed.

---

[148] Headache Classification Committee of the International Headache Society (IHS) The International Classification of Headache Disorders, 3rd edition. *Cephalalgia.* 2018;38(1):1-211. doi:10.1177/0333102417738202

Migraines

At least half the people who come into my office who say they have migraines don't have migraines but some other type of headache. Migraines make up only 10% of primary headaches. Tension-type headaches are about 4x more common and can mimic some migraine symptoms, particularly when more chronic. There are some features that are unique to migraines, some that aren't consistent with all migraines, and some that appear for all migraines but are common in other headaches too.[149] Migraines seem to have a genetic component and run in families. One defining feature of migraines is the difficulty to just "push through it." If you can just pop an Advil and still get your work done, you likely have a different type of headache. People who get migraines can also get tension-type headaches as well.

Migraines start with a trigger. People's triggers can vary: muscle pain, spicy food, caffeine, lack of sleep, medications, changes in the weather, changes in hormones, etc. There are 3-4 phases in the typical migraine once it is triggered.

The prodrome (or pre-headache) phase is where the brain/nervous system is ramping up in preparation to get over-excited during the main headache. This phase can last hours to days. The prodrome symptoms often involve the sympathetic and/or parasympathetic nervous systems. These are the fight/flight response and rest/digest systems of the body. The symptoms vary wildly between individuals. Some people never really figure out what their prodrome

---

[149] https://americanmigrainefoundation.org/

     BRANDON RAMAKKO

feels like. **Identifying the prodrome is extremely important in managing migraines.** Some common symptoms are fatigue, yawning, irritability, excitability, changes in energy, changes in mood, muscle stiffness, need to urinate, nausea, food cravings, difficulty speaking/reading, sensitivity to light or sound, eye dilation, sweating, itchiness, etc. Migraines are notoriously resistant to medications. Once the headache starts, then taking Excedrin, Tylenol, Advil, etc. isn't going to do anything. Even prescription medications have little to no effect on a migraine once it gets going. But in the prodrome phase, the migraine can be aborted! It can be frustrating as a migraine sufferer that nothing seems to help, but they likely have only tried solutions once the headache is already going. Aborting the migraine in the prodrome phase can be as simple as an over-the-counter pain reliever. For some, it might be as simple as using a hot or cold pack, taking a break, having a nap, staying hydrated, eating something, going to a quiet place, de-stressing, etc. Once you exit the prodrome phase, you'll just have to survive to the other side of the headache.

The second phase of the migraine often partially overlaps the prodrome phase and is called the "aura" phase. You can have migraines with aura or without. If you do get an aura, that is a more specific characteristic of migraines. But what is an "aura"? Like most things so far, it can vary between individuals, but it is a visual disturbance with stars, lights, shadows, colors, etc. This phase typically lasts 5 minutes to an hour.

Now we are at the main part of the headache. More often unilateral above or behind an eye. Most often described as throbbing, with sensitivity to light and/or sound, and with extreme resistance to medications. You need to just lie down until the headache is done. The headache phase lasts 4-72 hours.

The last phase is the postdrome phase. This is a migraine hangover. Since it isn't a particularly painful phase, it is poorly understood. Typical symptoms may be: feeling drained/tired/weary, aches, neck stiffness, brain fog, digestive issues, mild head pain/discomfort, hunger/thirst, mood changes, etc. Continuing the trend that everyone's symptoms could be different, some people feel euphoric or full of energy. The postdrome lasts 24 to 48 hours.

How to treat/manage migraines?

First, you can try to identify your triggers, and second, you can try to identify the signs of your prodrome. If these aren't obvious, you can keep a journal of how you are feeling and your actions. You may keep record of all your meals and snacks, looking for food triggers. Once your trigger is identified, you can avoid it (sadly, most people's triggers are work related). If you have identified your symptoms during the prodrome phase, you can start effectively treating it. Do not take headache relievers during a migraine headache; they have to be taken in the prodrome phase to work. Just a simple acetaminophen, Tylenol, Excedrin, Advil, ibuprofen can work. Just a massage or taking a long break or taking a nap can work. Find out what little thing you can do during the prodrome phase that can abort your migraine. I know two individuals who, if they get chiropractic adjustments during the prodrome phase, they won't get the full migraine.

Third, you can try medications/treatments between migraine attacks to lessen their frequency and/or severity. This may be Botox to the face, chiropractic adjustments, yoga, guided meditation, mental health counseling, massage, CoQ10, omega-3, diet changes, prescription meds, etc. I'll highlight CoQ10 and omega-3 supplementation. CoQ10 in most migraine sufferers reduces frequency of headaches by over 50% and seems to reduce intensity and duration as well.[150,151] The effects of omega-3 supplementation seems to be less consistent (probably depends on whether the sample population is deficient or not) but there are signs it helps with headache duration and perhaps intensity and frequency.[152,153] I will take a moment to mention that I have

---

[150] Shoeibi A, Olfati N, Soltani Sabi M, Salehi M, Mali S, Akbari Oryani M. Effectiveness of coenzyme Q10 in prophylactic treatment of migraine headache: an open-label, add-on, controlled trial. *Acta Neurol Belg.* 2017;117(1):103-109. doi:10.1007/s13760-016-0697-z

[151] Sazali S, Badrin S, Norhayati MN, Idris NS. Coenzyme Q10 supplementation for prophylaxis in adult patients with migraine-a meta-analysis. *BMJ Open.* 2021;11(1):e039358. Published 2021 Jan 5. doi:10.1136/bmjopen-2020-039358

[152] Maghsoumi-Norouzabad L, Mansoori A, Abed R, Shishehbor F. Effects of omega-3 fatty acids on the frequency, severity, and duration of migraine attacks: A systematic review and meta-analysis of randomized controlled trials. *Nutr Neurosci.* 2018;21(9):614-623. doi:10.1080/1028415X.2017.1344371

[153] Ramsden C E, Zamora D, Faurot K R, MacIntosh B, Horowitz M, Keyes G S et al. Dietary alteration of n-3 and n-6 fatty acids for headache reduction in adults with migraine: randomized controlled trial *BMJ* 2021; 374 :n1448 doi:10.1136/bmj.n1448

encountered those who have received some relief from Botox, but they all seemed to receive more relief through a thorough treatment of the jaw and neck muscles.

Tension-type Headaches

I'm going to cover tension-type headaches and myofascial trigger point pain referred to the head/face in the same section because they go together. It is rare to find one without the other or to differentiate them. Tension-type headaches are described as a pressing, tension-like, squeezing, achy pain. Most often described as a band around the head or starting at the back of the head then traveling to above the eye on one side or both sides. Tension-type headaches are cousins of the migraine and, when bad, they can mimic the symptoms of the migraine with throbbing and/or sensitivity to light or sound. Tension-type headaches normally are treatable to an extent. Muscle work to the neck or medication seems to help relieve the symptoms while a true migraine requires time, and nothing will help once it has started. Tension-type headaches you can push through, whereas with a true migraine, you can't.

Tension-type headaches are ultimately caused by the brain, but they have a close relationship to muscle pain, tightness, and discomfort in the neck, shoulder, and/or jaw. Imagine you are stressed (most of you don't have to imagine too hard), then you might be clenching your jaw or holding up your shoulders near your ears. If those muscles are tight long enough, then they will develop an achy soreness or full-on myofascial trigger points. The pain from the trigger points and achy muscles travels up the brainstem, which is more sensitive in tension-headache sufferers, which can cause the pain pattern on the sides of the head and forehead. If you treat the muscle pain or the stress, the headache often lessens. If you break the cycle by eliminating the muscle knots, then you can get rid of the headache. If you keep the muscle knots from reforming, then you may remain headache-free. It is very normal in my office for someone who gets chronic tension-type headaches (more than 15 days a month) to drop down to virtually no headaches (0-3 a month). Like everything, some people's cases are more challenging than others.

The images nearby show some of the common muscle knot locations. You can check out the jaw section for treatment of the jaw muscles.

Common Headache Muscle Knots 1

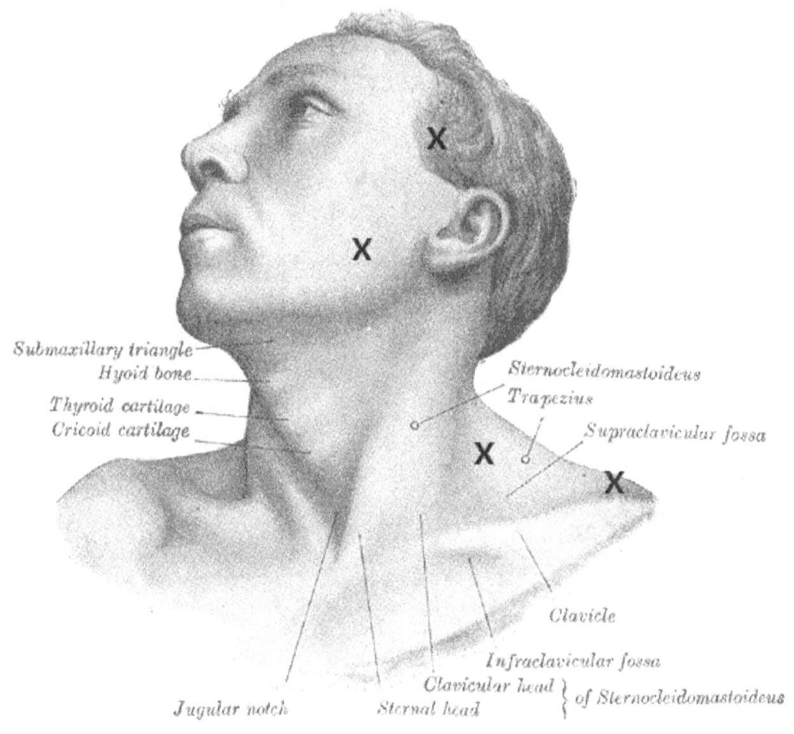

Common Headache Muscle Knots 2

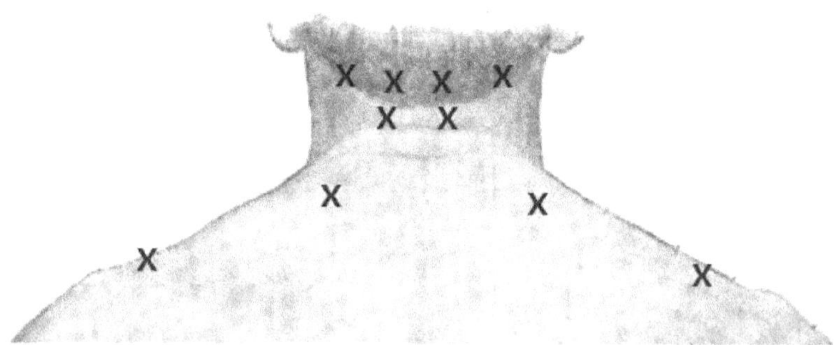

BRANDON RAMAKKO

Cervicogenic Headaches

The cervical region of the spine is the neck. The joints of the neck can cause headaches and dizziness/unsteadiness. This is much rarer than migraines and tension-type headaches. I find it often has overlap with tension-type headaches and/or muscle knot referred pain. This type of headache often occurs following a whiplash injury. It can persist until the neck is treated/rehabbed. If your headache is very sensitive to neck position, you have issues with unsteadiness, you have had a neck injury or history of neck pain, then this might be your type of headache. See the neck section of this book for more information since the problem comes from the neck, and once the neck is better, the headache will go away.

Chronic Post-Concussion Headaches

Post-concussion symptoms occur after a traumatic brain injury (TBI).[154] The initial headache post-concussion and other symptoms often resolve in 10-30 days for most. The initial headache (assuming no major brain bleeding) is caused by brain damage. The brain damage has to heal before anything else. Current recommendations, once brain bleeding is ruled out, is to rest and/or do gentle activities until you feel mostly better. This is a book on chronic problems, though, so let's dive into the chronic post-concussive

---

[154] Permenter CM, Fernández-de Thomas RJ, Sherman Al. Postconcussive Syndrome. [Updated 2022 Aug 29]. In: StatPearls [Internet]. Treasure Island (FL): *StatPearls Publishing*; 2023 Jan. Available from: https://www.ncbi.nlm.nih.gov/books/NBK534786/

issues. Common chronic symptoms are headache, fatigue, and dizziness/unsteadiness. There is a huge overlap with tension-type headaches and cervicogenic headaches. The treatment for chronic post-concussive headaches is sometimes more subtle and challenging compared to an average tension-type headache as the muscle knots involved are not the same. I can come across as pro-chiropractor in this book, but hopefully I'm more just pro-solution and I just happen to be more familiar with conservative treatments. I'll highlight the work of an MD, Dr. Phillip M. Steele, who uses ultrasound imaging to look for minor asymmetries in the deep muscles of the upper neck and uses mild anesthetic injections to improve symmetry and he gets reasonably good results. There is a whole subset of chiropractors who focus on just the upper neck, and some stubborn headache sufferers might get some relief there. Be cautious, as mentioned before, chiropractors might provide some relief, but it is easy to get into a pattern of dependence if they aren't combining their treatment with soft tissue work, balance exercises, eye exercises, and/or neuromuscular retraining. In particular, the muscles and fascia around the skull might play a role in symptoms, so "cranial techniques" might help. You have to remember that the initial brain injury has healed, and now you need to retrain your brain and/or body. How much retraining and exactly what type can vary person to person. If your eyes aren't behaving properly, then you have to retrain eye control. If moving your neck makes you unsteady/dizzy, then the information your neck is sending to the brain might be faulty, and you have to retrain that. Maybe the brain injury messed up your sense of where your feet are, and you have to just practice balancing with your eyes closed to regain a sense of where your feet are in space. Most commonly, in my experience, for chronic post-concussive symptoms, I treat them as if they have tension-headaches, have jaw problems, require neck rehab as if they have had whiplash, and I add in cranial techniques. I add in more specialized exercises as needed. They can respond so well to the passive treatments they can be resistant to doing the exercises, which are really hard/frustrating for them. Your brain doesn't want to do things it is bad at! But the exercises are the key to making the treatments last in a meaningful way.

Sinus Headaches

The sinuses are poorly understood by the majority of society. The skull has hollow chambers within it. Often pictures don't communicate their 3-dimensional nature. They produce mucus which makes its way to the nasal cavity (our nose). These sinus cavities are in our forehead, under and behind the eyes, and in our cheeks. If there is a build-up within a sinus, this can increase the pressure, resulting in a headache, normally directly above the sinus location. Chronic sinus issues can be related to allergies and/or a blockage.

If this blockage is a polyp (a physical growth/non-cancerous tumor) within the lining of the sinus, then CT imaging will be able to identify it, and then it can be removed surgically. If the issue is something else wrong with the opening to the sinus, then the opening may be surgically widened. A balloon may even be inflated within the sinus cavity to treat the lining within the sinus and help with drainage. Seeing an ear-nose-throat (ENT) doctor would be a typical first step to this solution.

Do all sinus problems require surgery?

No, even if there are polyps, they might not be causing your problems and plenty of people have problems without polyps.

Are there treatments for non-polyp related chronic congestion/post-nasal drip/sinus headaches?

Yes. First, some more anatomy. The nasal cavity itself is divided into 3 connected regions/spaces on each side. So, in addition to the 8 sinuses which drain into the nasal cavity, we have 6 spaces within the nasal cavity. Chronic problems are an irritation problem and/or a drainage problem. What can we do without surgery?

One option is cranial techniques and/or acupressure points: gentle but firm force is applied to the bones of the skull. This pressure seems to be able to alleviate congestion symptoms or headaches in some individuals. There are some points in the face directly related to their nearby sinus and there are cranial moves that involve a more shearing force across the skull. Some practitioners erroneously say they are moving the bones of the skull, and it can even feel that way with how the pressure seems to release, but the joints of the skull are firm fibrous joints which eventually calcify as we age. See the nearby images for the common pressure points and one common shearing force procedure to try. Normally you can feel a difference in how easy it is to breath after a breath or two. If you feel relief, try it for 10 breaths and see how long the relief lasts. Sadly, this relief seems to be more temporary, but if it is effective for you, use it as much as you want. Instead of pressure, acupuncture needles may also be used. This type of treatment can be done by osteopaths, chiropractors, physiotherapists, massage therapists, naturopaths, or acupuncturists, but they might not all be trained in such a procedure, so call in advance.

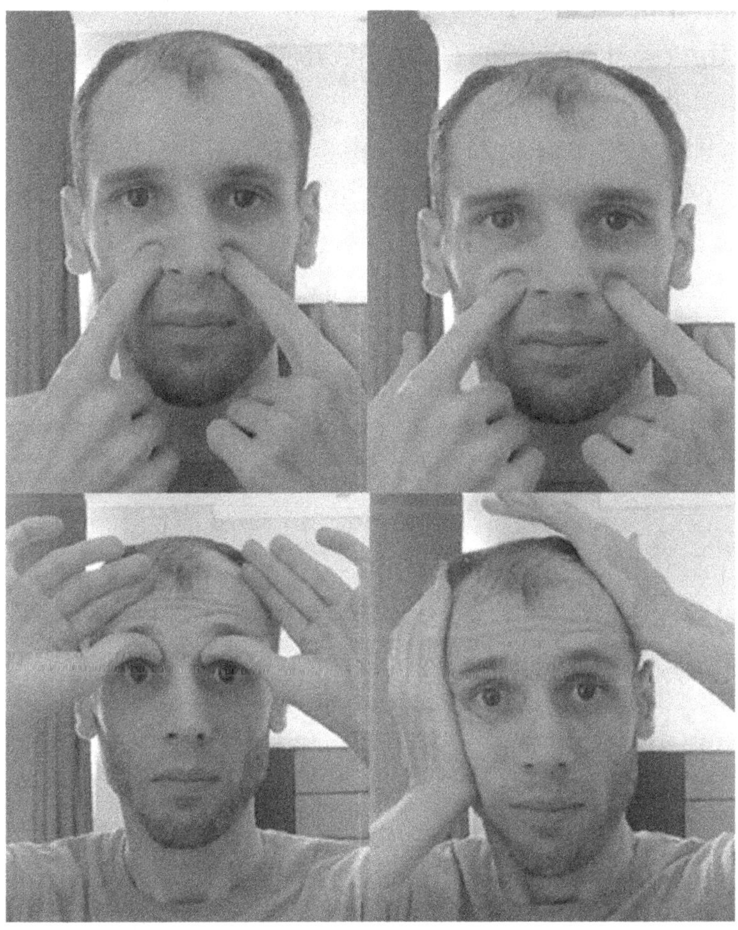

Another type of treatment is called nasal specific, but there are similar treatments by slightly different names. The commonality is that they all involve placing a small balloon into the nasal cavity and inflating it quickly. This might seem very similar to a surgical procedure where a medical doctor inserts a balloon into a sinus that requires widening of the opening between the sinus and the nasal cavity. Frustratingly, they will do the more extreme version but won't use the balloon treatment for the nasal cavity. While a balloon into the nose won't help a polyp in the sinus, I've found approximately 80% of my patients experience significant relief with this technique. Chiropractors and osteopaths have been using this technique for decades. My theory is that it helps loosen any physical blockage that might be affecting the drainage into the nasal cavity. It also massages all the soft tissue within the cavity. Some chiropractors claim it works by moving/shifting and/or loosening the bones of the skull. Some claim the benefit is from improved cerebral spinal fluid flow due to improved joint motion between cranial bones, but there is virtually no support for this explanation. I think the pressure mechanically affecting the lining of the nasal cavity in such a way that normal drainage of the sinuses can resume is more likely.

Another possible, non-surgical treatment is by using Argyrol: an anti-septic (anti-microbial) chemical. Some of it is placed on a Q-tip which is then inserted into the middle cavity of the nose which stimulates the drainage of the connected sinuses. The recommended treatment is 1-3 sessions within about a week's time. Each treatment takes about 20-30 minutes. Nothing happens for the first 5 minutes, and then the drainage will start. This is normally performed by a naturopath, but osteopaths or chiropractors might be familiar with it.

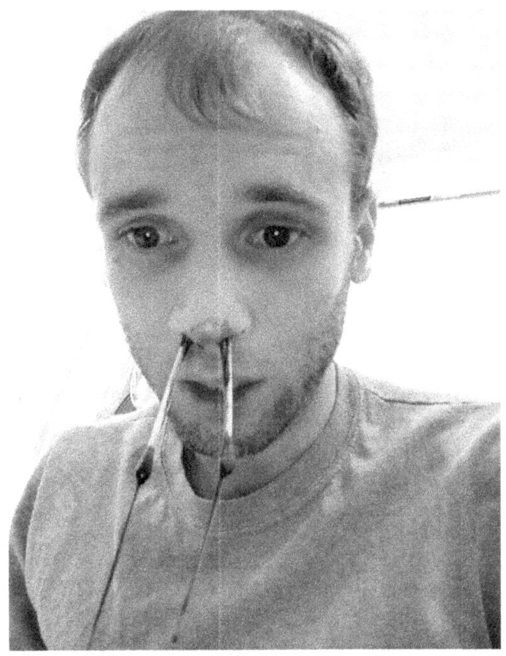

PRESSURE IN THE EAR

Pressure in the ear can be related to causes of chronic dizziness since the balance organs are kept in that region but can also be unrelated. For loss of hearing and/or room spinning sensations, see the dizziness section of the book. If the only symptom is ear pressure or ear popping, this issue can be fluid persisting in the ear from an infection. To improve drainage of the ear, the eustachian tube must be opened. This tube connects the inner ear to the back of the nose/throat. The nasal specific treatment covered in the last section may be enough to push on the involved tissues. A physician, naturopath, osteopath, or chiropractor may try to reach to the back of the throat and upwards to release/relax the muscles which control the tube's opening which can allow for drainage. If the ear fullness is changed by neck rotations, then working on the muscles of the upper neck (particularly on the front) and the jaw can sometimes provide resolution/relief.

TINNITUS

Tinnitus is the ringing in your ears, particularly prominent after being exposed to very loud sounds, causing hearing damage. Get your hearing checked if you have tinnitus. Sometimes a hearing aid or white noise machines can help. If it has come on recently without loud sounds as a cause, particularly if vertigo/dizziness is involved, please seek a doctor for evaluation. Some types of tinnitus vary in intensity with neck motion, and if the neck is treated/rehabbed, the tinnitus can be reduced in intensity.[155]

---

[155] Sanchez TG, Rocha CB. Diagnosis and management of somatosensory tinnitus: review article. *Clinics* (Sao Paulo). 2011;66(6):1089-1094. doi:10.1590/s1807-59322011000600028

DIZZINESS

There are different types of dizziness: a sense of spinning/movement, unsteadiness, and lightheadedness. The causes can be even more varied. There are 2 scenarios that are easily treated conservatively: benign paroxysmal positional vertigo (BPPV) and cervicogenic dizziness, which are the two we'll cover.

Benign paroxysmal positional vertigo (BPPV) happens when small crystals/stones make their way into the inner ear apparatus which detects head movement (semicircular canals). When your head moves, the motion of the stones causes a sensation of continued motion which lasts 10-15s before the stones settle again. By putting the head through a sequence of positions, it is possible to coax the stones to leave the canal, thereby eliminating symptoms. The most typical set of positions is called the Epley maneuver which targets the canal with the highest likelihood of having crystals in it. There are two other sets of movements which are less commonly required, that may be necessary if you have crystals in one of the other two canals. BPPV has a fairly distinct set of symptoms: the symptoms can be reproduced with head movement, the symptoms last less than a minute, and the sensation is of spinning movement. There are no associated hearing symptoms with this condition. It can happen to anyone, but the risk factors for this condition are: being a woman, vitamin D deficiency, osteoporosis, migraines, head trauma, and high total cholesterol.[156]

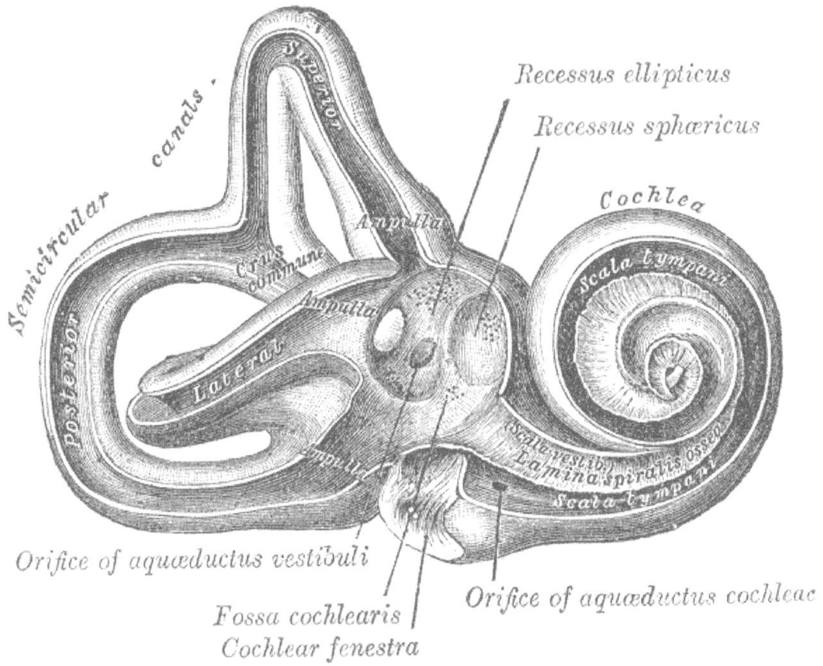

Cervicogenic dizziness is dizziness/unsteadiness caused by the neck. Neck position and movement information is sent to the brainstem along with visual information from the eyes and balance/movement information from the inner ear. If there is a disagreement in the information, it can affect your sense of balance and eye coordination. A neck injury can result in faulty information being sent to the brainstem, which can be the cause of the symptoms and a

---

[156] Chen J, Zhao W, Yue X, Zhang P. Risk Factors for the Occurrence of Benign Paroxysmal Positional Vertigo: A Systematic Review and Meta-Analysis. *Front Neurol.* 2020;11:506. Published 2020 Jun 23. doi:10.3389/fneur.2020.00506

chiropractor/physiotherapist can help by mobilizing and/or rehabbing the neck. Symptoms are often worse in the evenings when the brain is tired.

There is another type of unsteadiness which is basically lack of practice. Our capabilities shrink over time to what we do every day. If the variety is limited, then our body forgets what to do. I remember one case where an older gentleman, early 80s, complained that he kept on falling over. After visiting a neurologist, they concluded there was nothing wrong with him. He also did all the balance exercises he could find on YouTube or assigned by physiotherapists to his friends. But still he lost his balance every now and then. When I checked his balance using the standard tests, he had no balance issues, but he had practiced those tests. He could easily stand on one leg for 60 seconds because he was practicing it every day. I then asked him what the scenario was where he last fell, and we tried to replicate it in my office. It was twisting and reaching for the shelves above his sink, and I had to catch him from falling over. We practiced that and we practiced getting in and out of the car. We even practiced these movements while I was randomly shoving him. If he can hold his balance when I randomly push him, then he should be able to maintain his balance under normal conditions! It only took maybe 4-6 visits before he said he finally felt confident in his balance again.

NECK

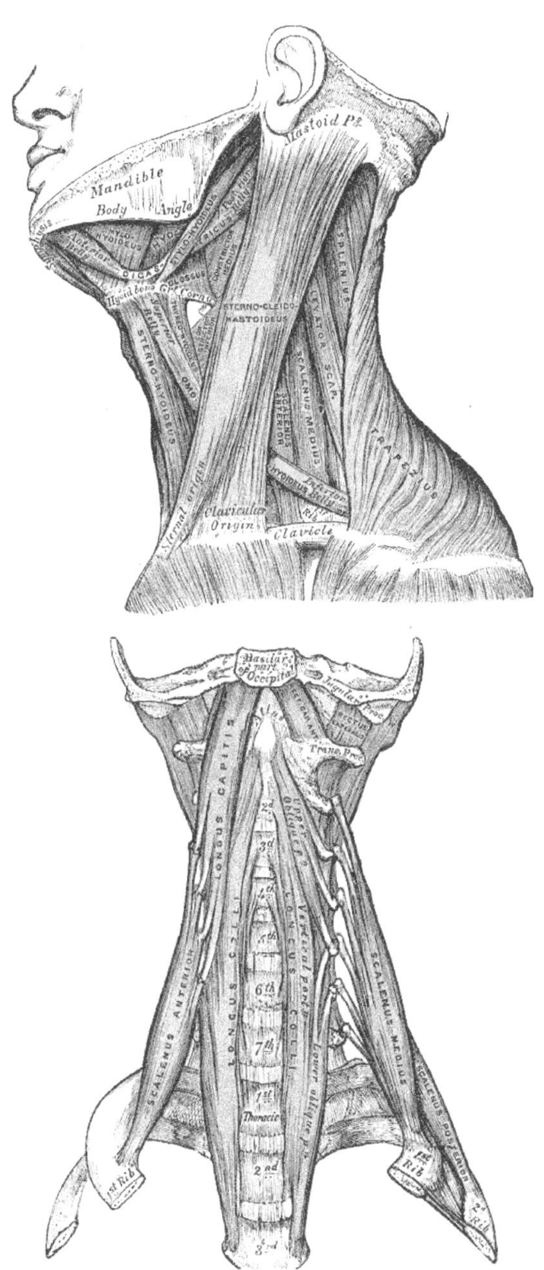

Mastoid Pt.
Mandible
Body
Angle
STERNO-CLEIDO-MASTOIDEUS
SPLENIUS
LEVATOR SCAP.
SCALENUS MEDIUS
STERNO-HYOIDEUS
TRAPEZIUS
Sternal origin
Clavicular Origin
Clavicle
Basilar part
of Occipita
LONGUS CAPITIS
LONGUS COLLI
SCALENUS ANTERIOR
SCALENUS MEDIUS
SCALENUS POSTERIOR
1st Rib
2nd Rib
3rd

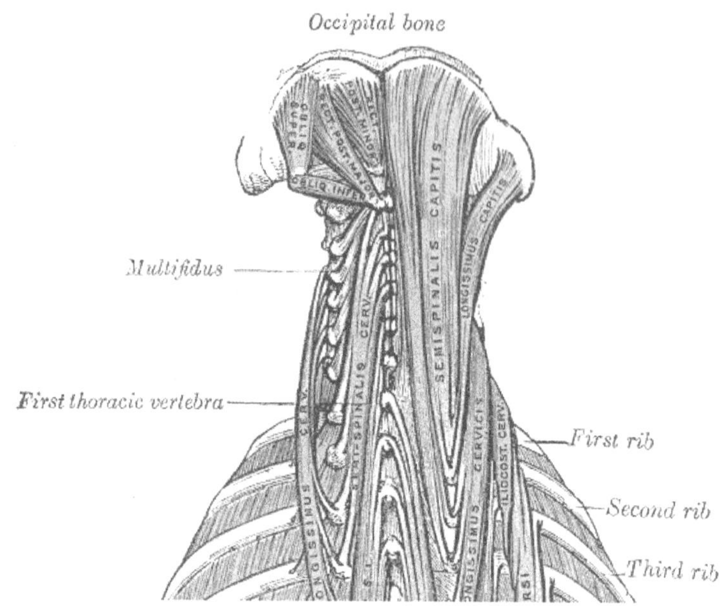

Neck pain can be closely related to headaches, jaw pain, ear pressure, dizziness, shoulder pain, arm pain, and hand pain, so check those sections as well. First, let's start talking about the anatomy of the neck.

Functionally, you could argue the whole spine acts together, but more specifically, neck motion involves the skull (labeled C0), the vertebrae of the neck (labeled C1-C7), and the top few vertebrae of the back (labeled T1-T4). The top vertebrae are very unique. The top vertebrae have a different set of muscles and a different shape. This region of the neck is often implicated in cervicogenic headaches, tension-type headaches, whiplash pain, and unsteadiness more so than any other. C1 is a ring and C2 has a bony protrusion sticking out the top that C1 makes contact with. C1 can rotate around this bony prominence. Most of your neck's rotation comes from just this joint. C1 is called the atlas because it holds up the world (your head) and C2 is called the axis

                                                BRANDON RAMAKKO

(that your head rotates on). T1-T4 are more rigid in general due to being attached to ribs 1-4. Most vertebrae of the neck look and work the same and are similar to vertebrae in the rest of the spine: there are two joints on either side, near the back, and there is a disc in the front separating the vertebral bodies. There are bony protrusions out the back (spinous processes) and out the sides (transverse processes) that act as attachment points for the muscles. As for muscles, let's break them into 5 parts. The Scalene muscles are long muscles that attach from the upper ribs to the upper neck. There are 3 of them: anterior, middle, and posterior. The anterior and middle may be implicated in nerve pain, tingling, and numbness and/or office work stiffness. The posterior scalenes, more than the others, can be chronically and protectively tight in chronic neck pain conditions and/or post car-accident. I often use these muscles to gauge how well someone's neck rehab is going. If I stretch it and it is tight 30 minutes later, we need more rehab, and if it takes more than a week to tighten up significantly, then we are likely done rehab. The sternocleidomastoid (SCM) muscle goes from the front clavicle region to the skull behind the ear. The levator scapulae muscle connects the shoulder blade (scapula) to the upper neck. If you think about it, how does the shoulder blade attach to the rest of the body? How does it transfer the weight of your arms to your spine? While they do lean on the ribs, the muscles that connect the shoulder to the upper neck directly transfers the load. So, if you are lifting something heavy with your arms, you are basically lifting that thing with your neck! Neck muscles are surprisingly strong. Next are the muscles along the spinous processes. These tend to get a little tight and achy but otherwise don't bother people. The muscles along the front of the neck can be troublesome in chronic pain patients. These muscles may be disused, discoordinated, and atrophied. You can't see or easily feel these muscles as they are deep, behind your esophagus and trochlea (throat and windpipe). The last group of muscles is the suboccipital muscles. The occiput is the part of the lower back of the skull, so suboccipital means underneath the occiput, which is the top of the neck. The muscles and joints here are most associated with headaches and unsteadiness. The muscle knots for neck pain can be similar to those for tension-type headaches, so see the images in that section for their location.

Let's focus on the joints of the neck. These joints are called the zygapophyseal or facet joints. Over time, these joints form bone spurs/spikes at their edges. These bony changes are normally the ones noticed when they tell someone they have osteoarthritis in their neck. I'll remind you that these are normal age-related bony changes and have a poor correlation to pain. There is some correlation to pain, but there is also correlation with bad posture, bad movement habits, and chronically tight muscles. If your neck muscles are chronically tight on both sides of your neck, then this would result in more pressure on these joints. Also, when your head is jutting forward, like a turtle, these joints are more in contact. This could explain the increased bony changes/arthritis. These joints are synovial joints. Synovial joints are joints that are filled with fluid. So, there is a sac that contains the fluid. This sac is incredibly painful if pinched. The medical terminology for this is synovial fold/meniscoid impingement/entrapment/extrapment. Any pain related to these joints could be called a "facet syndrome."

Another part of the spine is the disc. Disc herniations and bulges are rarer in the neck than the low back but can occur. They are also found in asymptomatic patients as well. The treatment for disc issues of the neck and the low back are similar, so see the low back section for more information. In short, there are particular exercises that may relieve disc-related pain called Makenzie or directional preference exercises. Depending on how the disc is injured, the motion that is relieving might be different. Since this book is about chronic problems and not acute/fresh injuries, we won't talk too much about disc pain here, as most people who have had a disc injury of the neck develop a type of chronic neck pain similar to those with other neck injuries despite assuming that "it's that old disc herniation acting up again."

While there can be different acute neck problems, like a car accident causing ligament and muscle tears, a synovial fold pinch, or a disc herniation, what causes the problem to become chronic can be similar in all cases. When you injure the neck, you don't move the neck properly for a few days to a few weeks. Your brain forgets how to coordinate the tiny muscles for fine motor control of the neck and starts relying on the larger muscles (scalenes, levator scap) to move your neck. It may even start to keep both sides of your neck tight as a protective mechanism. Eventually, you turn your neck too quickly or are pulling your neck straight first thing in the morning and the joint slips/buckles and pinches the facet joints. The body can go into panic mode. The pain system kicks into high gear, making moving painful even if little to no damage occurred. You will recover, but this will start happening more and more often and you'll have a chronically tight and achy neck, likely with tension-type headaches from your long neck muscles being tight 100% of the time. You may develop the central sensitization I talked about at the beginning of this book. You will fear moving in case you throw out your neck again.

The solution?

Recondition the atrophied muscles and retrain the brain's control of the neck. Plus, eliminate muscle knots and improve posture habits.

How to tell if neck rehab is right for you?

If I just stretch out someone's tight muscles of the neck, they often will tighten up by the next day... sometimes by the end of the visit! The brain wants those muscles to stay tight to protect the neck, so if I relax them, the brain says, "Why did you relax those? I'm using them!" and tightens back up. These individuals report that getting a massage doesn't help at all. In fact, sometimes I relax the large neck muscles, and if the muscle coordination isn't there and we haven't done enough rehab, the joints buckle that day after the session and it triggers a crick in the neck. I always try to do exercises with these individuals when I relax muscles to make sure the muscles are awake and ready to control the newly relaxed and flexible neck. People who require this type of rehab can also be identified by their eyes and ability to balance. Sometimes a deconditioned neck sends faulty information to the brain. Since all the other balance organs are in the brain, if the brain can't figure out where the body is in relation to the head, then that leads to a feeling of unsteadiness. Particularly worse in the evenings when the brain is tired. When my neck was bad, if I tried to walk with my head tilted to one side, I would immediately fall over! When you tell your eyes to track an object, the eye muscles will use the information from the neck to figure out what to do. A test called gaze stability checks this. I have a patient stare at a single point and have them painfully slowly turn their head as they stare at it. Their eyes might dart back and forth (called saccades) indicating that the eye slides off the object and had to manually readjust. The patient reports/interprets this as blurry vision. Another sign they need rehab during the test is if their neck moves like clockwork with jitters and start-stop type motion. This is an indication the fine motor control of the neck is bad. A final test I often use is to check how weak the fine motor control muscles have become. If I have them set up with their head unsupported but with their head back and chin tucked, then the large muscles can't help, and the small muscles will be tested (Jull's test). A healthy and strong neck should be able to reach approximately 60 seconds. Averages are normally around 30 seconds.[157] Most of the people who need rehab can't reach 10 seconds.

Pinched Nerves

A sharp pain associated with waking up with a kink in the neck is more likely to be facet joint pain than a compressed nerve. The pain from the joints and discs can refer to the shoulder blade regions and over the shoulders. Shoulder muscle knots can refer pain all the way down to the hand, so if you have neck pain plus shoulder muscle knots, that

---

[157] Domenech MA, Sizer PS, Dedrick GS, McGalliard MK, Brismee JM. The deep neck flexor endurance test: normative data scores in healthy adults. *PM R.* 2011;3(2):105-110. doi:10.1016/j.pmrj.2010.10.023

can mimic nerve pain down to the hand. Tingling and/or numbness are more specific to nerve issues than pain is. Lack of feeling and muscle weakness is very specific to nerve issues. With significant weakness, you should let a health professional know, and an MRI should be ordered. If there is no significant weakness, surgery is rarely performed, and MRI is normally uncalled for. The spinal cord could be compressed (more dangerous) affecting both sides and/or both lower and upper body, or, much more commonly, the nerve roots could be compressed. Neck position combined with osteophytes (bone spurs) can compress the nerve roots as they are exiting the spinal cord through openings between the vertebrae. The osteophytes grow as people age, so it can become more of an issue later in life. If you have neck pain plus grip weakness, that could be nerve root compression at the neck (radiculopathy) but it could also be neck pain plus nerve compression at the shoulder, forearm, and/or wrist. People are allowed to have more than one problem which can make diagnosis and targeting treatment challenging. In fact, nerves can be compressed at multiple locations, making you think one location was the problem because you improved a bit when that region was worked on, but then your status plateaus, and your clinician/therapist needs to revisit the other regions where the nerve could be compressed. This is why I stressed earlier in this book that if your therapist is not re-evaluating and/or modifying treatment when progress is stalling, it is a sign of a bad therapist. When treating a cervical radiculopathy (neck nerve root compression), I now check the other places the nerve could be compressed regularly.

Disc Pain

Disc injury can lead to nerve or spinal cord compression. The pain from the disc itself can spread. The pain is very sharp and can lock up the neck. It can take months to resolve, if it does entirely. What do I mean by "entirely"? Well, the disc doesn't repair perfectly. If a later MRI is taken, the disc might not look 100% like normal. But pain from the disc often does resolve within a month or two. Most people's pain later in life after a disc injury, is facet joint (not disc) and is caused by lack of rehab as explained earlier in this chapter. That is great news!

If you do injure a disc or are one of the few that does get true recurring disc pain, one treatment which is particularly effective for discs is called the "Makenzie protocol" or its no-name alternative "directional preference." To put it simply, the treatment involves finding a motion that, when repeated, centralizes the pain (pain spreads less) and/or improves range of motion. This may be flexion (chin to chest), extension (looking up), rotations, lateral flexions (ear to shoulder), retraction (double chin), or protraction (sticking chin out). Finding out which direction works can require a bit of experimentation. If any of the directions, when repeated 10 times, works, then you repeat the treatment every hour until you fully recover from the disc issue. If I think it is a disc, I often start with trying to find the motion that helps. If it does help and they feel better without me doing anything, and that is for the best. I don't have to ask them to do the exercise because they associate feeling better with the exercise. This exercise is an all-natural and effective "pain-killer" during recovery. I used to do electrical stim and neck mobilizations, but if that helped them, then they are less convinced to try the exercises and more likely to become reliant on passive care (good for making me money but not the most ethical).

How to rehab the neck?

Regardless of how the neck is injured and what the injured structure was, rehab exercises can look approximately the same. If the deep fine motor control muscles have atrophied (weakened), I like starting with strengthening them. The way to test this is something called Jull's test (there are other tests too). Place a pillow underneath your shoulders lying on a yoga mat on the floor. You want your shoulders to be slightly higher than where the back of your head would be. Then you try to hold your head in-line with your body with the chin tucked as long as possible. If the head moves higher or the chin doesn't stay tucked, that is a fail. Ideally, you can do more than 20 seconds. Less than 10 seconds or a complete inability indicates extreme weakness of these muscles. You are guaranteed to have a lifetime of pain unless you get these muscles working again. This test can be turned into an exercise such as 2 sets of 5x5 seconds. These muscles might be so weak that exercises can't be done every day because the muscles are sore. That is okay. The muscles need time to heal. Bodybuilders don't work out the same muscle groups every day. Instead of a hold, you may prefer to raise the head up and down (while keeping the chin tucked). Another variation is to do these exercises reclined so you aren't working against the full force of gravity. You could also do it sitting upright using your hand to provide the force that gravity normally would. This has the advantage of giving you control of the amount of force.

If you move the neck, there are likely jitters when trying to go slowly. If you practice the jittery motion, eventually you will retrain the neck to move smoothly again. This can go quickly. and may only take a few days for some, but you have to make sure you retrain all possible neck motions! You can start with working on one or two, and then as they get better, find new motions that are jittery or where you find your neck doesn't do exactly what you tell it to (doing a diagonal often turns into stair steps). Some people mount laser pointers to their heads and try to write on the wall or draw shapes. Be careful to train your neck in a more neutral position. If you practice with your head jutting out like a turtle, then that is where your neck is going to stay. This is brain training so it can be done daily, multiple times, as it doesn't really tire out the muscles, just the brain. I find these exercises hard to do for more than a minute at a time before my brain gets tired.

Your neck should have the capacity to adapt to an external force. Try the exercises from the last paragraph while lying on your side or on all fours. Different, right? Variety here is also key to making your neck more robust. Use gravity or your hand to provide the force and use a variety of neck motions.

Throughout rehab, working out muscle knots or loosening the neck may help as it may reduce pain and improve range of motion. So, a chiropractor, physiotherapist, or acupuncturist may help with this. There is a useful at-home segmental stretch of the cervical (neck) segments of the spine called sustained natural apophyseal glides (SNAGs). You basically use the edge of a hand towel to add a little overpressure at a particular segment in the neck as you either rotate the neck or look upwards. Afterwards, the towel can be moved upwards and/or downwards to target other individual segments. A pin-and-stretch of the anterior scalenes might also help. Keep in mind, the relief from stretching won't stick unless you do the exercises!

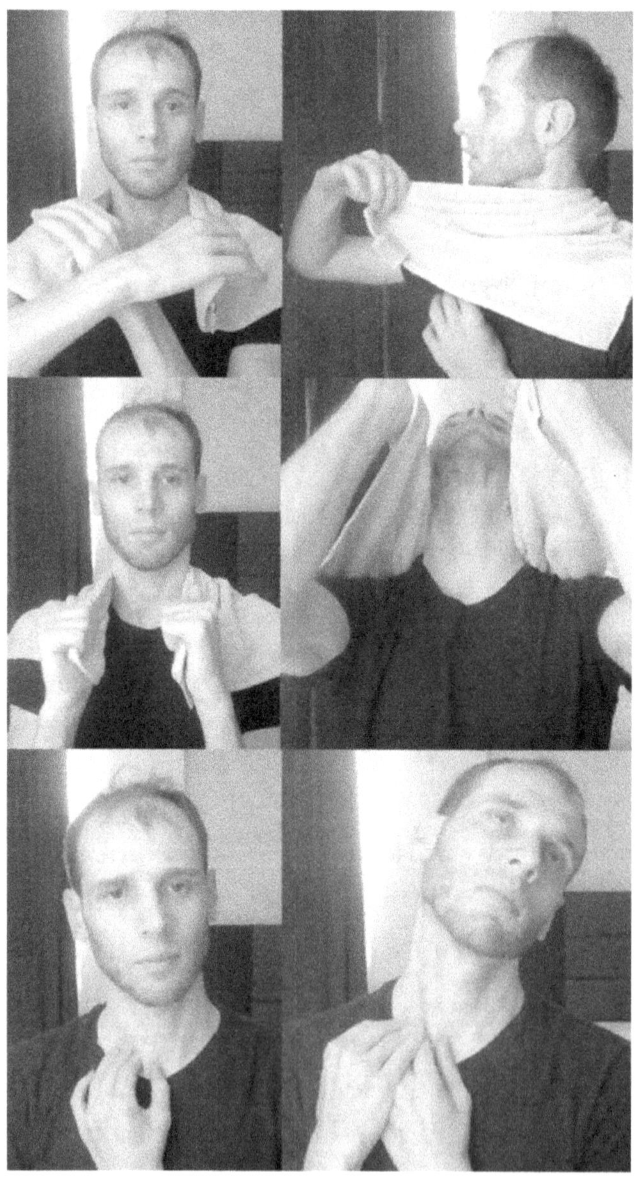

NOTE: Those with congenital abnormalities, surgical fusions, rheumatoid arthritis, and down syndrome should let the practitioner know. In particular, those with rheumatoid arthritis should not let chiropractors, physiotherapists, or osteopaths crack the top of the neck. They can use the clicker though.

JAW (TMJ)

Temporal bone
Zygomatic process
Mandible

Mandib. fossa
Articular tubercle
SYNOVIAL CAVITY
ARTICULAR DISC.
SYNOVIAL CAVITY
ARTICULAR
Condyle
PTERYGOIDEUS EXTERNUS

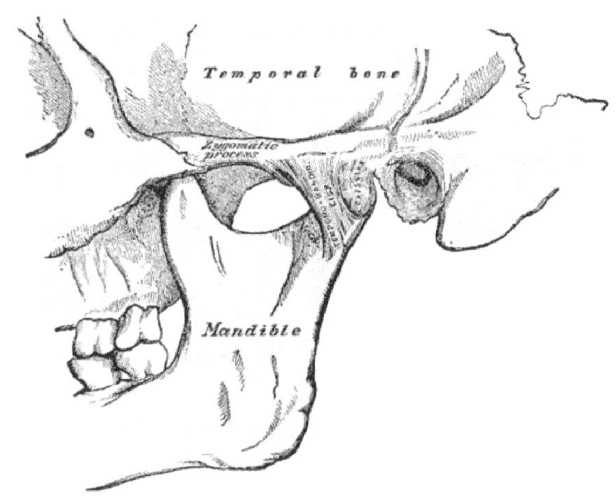

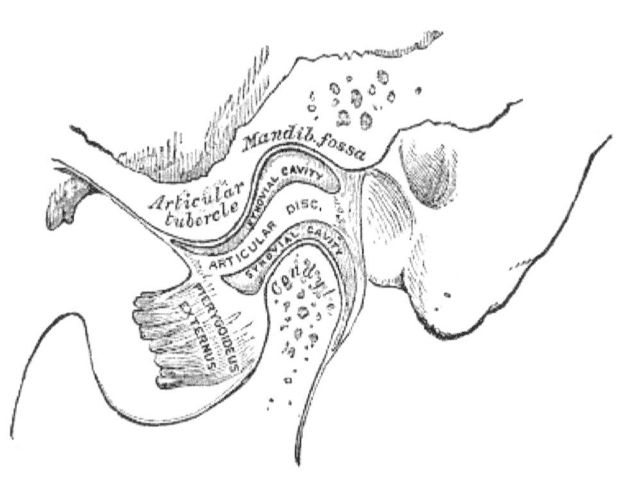

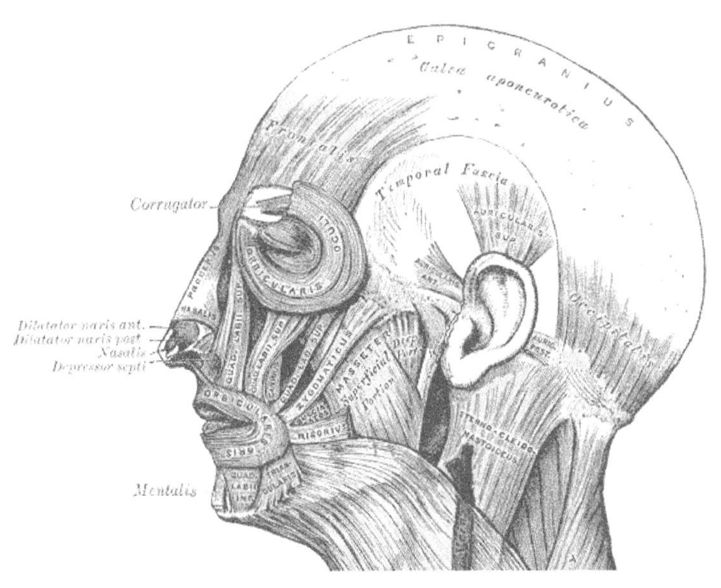

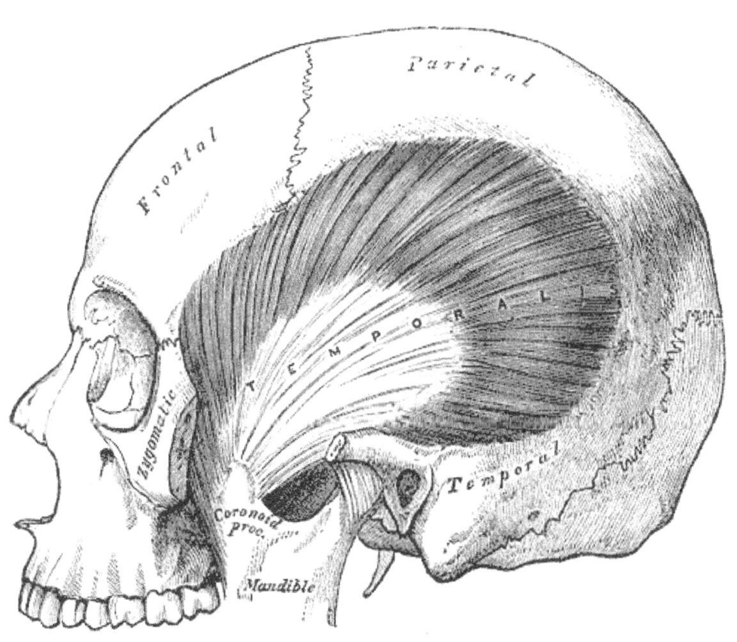

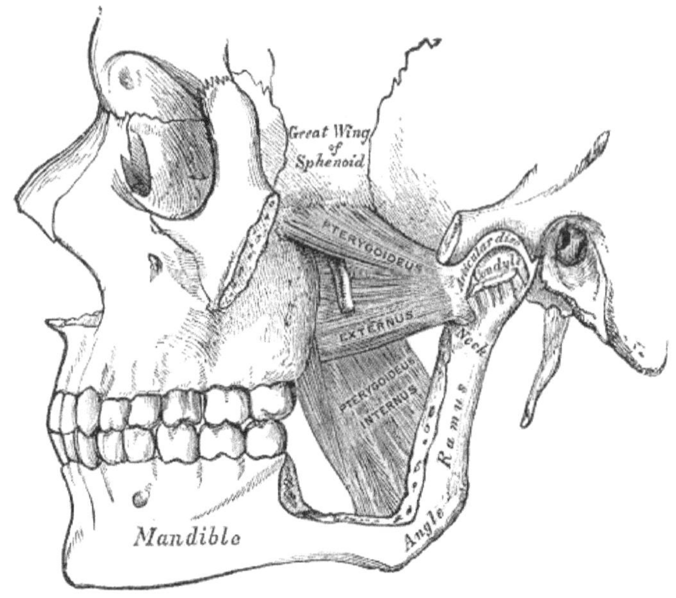

The joint of the jaw is quite interesting. Each joint is actually two joints, or you can imagine it as an elongated joint with two articulation points. As you start to open your mouth, the jaw rotates, then the jaw slides forward as you open it more, and the joint slides onto the lower/frontal joint surface, where the last bit of rotation happens. There is a disc between the jaw and the skull that actually slides from one point of rotation to the other. The movement is coordinated by multiple muscles including the temporalis (at your temples) and the masseter (near the back of your cheek). A loud click could be the jaw sliding on and/or off of the disc. The name of the joint is the Temporomandibular Joint (TMJ). I have patients that come in all the time saying they have TMJ. We all have TMJ, we all have two of them! The correct medical term for a problem with the joint would be TMJ pain, TMJ disorder, or TMJ dysfunction.

Problems in the jaw can vary wildly: tension, popping/clicking, grinding/crepitus, limited opening of the jaw, locking, tenderness, jaw deviating to one side, etc. Treatment might vary depending on the presentation but normally involves treating tender or tight muscles to try to relax tension, and exercises to improve the coordination of the muscles. A chiropractic "adjustment" (using a special adjustment tool, clicker/activator, set to one of its gentlest settings) might also be indicated. Treating the neck (particularly the upper neck) is also a best practice when addressing a jaw issue, because an upper neck issue can cause pain and/or interfere with muscle control of the jaw.[158,159] The jaw issues might come back without jaw and/or neck rehab.

So, I should see my dentist, right?

You can if you want, but sadly and confusingly, dentists are not trained to treat jaw joint/muscle dysfunction. The one tool they have at their disposal is night guards/splints. If you only have a hammer, every problem looks like a nail. Since it is a muscle and joint problem, a chiropractor or physiotherapist trained in TMJ pain is a better choice.

---

[158] Sanchla AD, Shrivastav S, Bharti L, Kamble R. Comparative Evaluation and Correlation of Pain Pattern in Neck Musculature Observed in Mild, Moderate, and Severe Temporomandibular Joint Disorder Cases as Compared to Non-temporomandibular Joint Disorder Cases. *Cureus.* 2022;14(10):e30099. Published 2022 Oct 9. doi:10.7759/cureus.30099

[159] Ana Izabela S. de Oliveira-Souza, Josepha Karinne de O. Ferro, Manuella M.M.B. Barros, Daniella A. de Oliveira, Cervical musculoskeletal disorders in patients with temporomandibular dysfunction: A systematic review and meta-analysis, *Journal of Bodywork and Movement Therapies*, Volume 24, Issue 4, 2020, Pages 84-101, ISSN 1360-8592, https://doi.org/10.1016/j.jbmt.2020.05.001.

Do night guards help at all?

Sometimes. The primary goal of a night guard is to protect your teeth from being damaged from grinding. Some report improvements in muscle tension as well. Overall, getting your muscles treated is more effective.[160]

How to treat the muscle in the Jaw?

There are four muscles of mastication that are normally treated, two on the outside and two on the inside of the mouth. The outside ones respond well to massage and pin-and-stretch stretch for tightness. They can have tender spots that can refer to pain to the face. Ischemic compression works best for these. The internal muscles are very tender when mad but relax surprisingly quickly, normally within 10 seconds of pressure.

 What are jaw exercises like?

There is a large variety of jaw exercises just like there is for the shoulder, knee, or ankle. Some focus on control, such as looking in a mirror practicing using the muscles to keep the jaw straight during slow opening and closing. Some focus on exercising certain muscle groups by using resistance or by practicing moving the jaw in different directions: opening, closing, lateral glides to each side, retraction towards the throat, and protraction protruding away from your face.

---

[160] Kapos FP, Exposto FG, Oyarzo JF, Durham J. Temporomandibular disorders: a review of current concepts in aetiology, diagnosis and management. *Oral Surg.* 2020;13(4):321-334. doi:10.1111/ors.12473

SHOULDER

The shoulder joint is the most unstable joint in the body.[161] It has an insane amount of mobility as it can move and rotate in so many ways. The joint is often described as a golf ball on a golf tee. As the joint can do so much, it requires many muscles to coordinate the motion of this joint, and each muscle plays multiple roles, which can depend on the position of the arm. If the muscle coordination is bad, it can result in pops, clicks, and irritation/pain. If we limit ourselves just to muscles that cross the joint, then we have the rotator cuff muscles: supraspinatus, infraspinatus, subscapularis, and teres minor; and then the other muscles: deltoid, pec major, teres major, latissimus dorsi, coracobrachialis, biceps, and triceps. This doesn't even include the muscles that control the scapula (shoulder blade) such as the levator scapulae, trapezius, and rhomboids. Coordination of the shoulder blade is arguably just as important as the shoulder joint. Most shoulder blade muscles attach to the spine and neck.

Relearning muscle coordination is an essential part of recovering from any shoulder injury and is necessary in

---

[161] Cuéllar R, Ruiz-Ibán MA, Cuéllar A. Anatomy and Biomechanics of the Unstable Shoulder. *Open Orthop J.* 2017;11:919-933. Published 2017 Aug 31. doi:10.2174/1874325001711010919

resolving virtually all chronic pain conditions of the shoulder. The longer the pain has gone on, the more rehab that may be necessary.

The shoulder is an area that is prone to central sensitization and chronic pain syndromes. There are many more nerve sensors located at the top of the shoulder to inform the brain when the shoulder isn't moving right. It can be confusing for radiologists because someone can have pain in one shoulder but when both shoulders are imaged, they look the same. You can also have two virtually identical MRI's or ultrasounds showing degeneration or injury, and one patient will have little to no pain while the other may have debilitating pain. Pain and/or disability levels don't necessarily correlate well with pathology seen on imaging, particularly on older individuals (with more degenerative/deconditioned pathologies). Asymptomatic (non-painful) rotator cuff tears have a prevalence somewhere between 8-40% in the general adult population (with increased prevalence in the elderly).[162]

The pain could be from the neck!

The neck can send pain to the shoulder. The discs and facet joints in the cervical spine can refer pain to the shoulder region. Also, if the nerves are compressed, that can cause pain/tingling/weakness in the shoulder, forearm, and/or hands. If you move your neck and you feel it affect the arm or hands, chances are some or all of your shoulder problems are coming from the neck region. Weakness is specific to

---

[162] Lawrence RL, Moutzouros V, Bey MJ. Asymptomatic Rotator Cuff Tears. *JBJS* Rev. 2019;7(6):e9. doi:10.2106/JBJS.RVW.18.00149

nerve issues, but pain could be nerves, muscles, discs, or facet joints of the neck.

There is one nerve impingement issue that can occur right at the neck/shoulder, and it can be more chronic/annoying. This issue is called thoracic outlet syndrome (TOS). The nerves come out of the neck then travel under the clavicle and under the pec muscles to get to the arm. The nerves can be pinched under the pecs or between the clavicle and the ribs. I'm mentioning it here, but this type of issue normally results in hand symptoms more than shoulder symptoms. In fact, some people who think they have carpal tunnel syndrome often have TOS. Sometimes TOS can be caused by extra ribs which can be removed surgically or by a tumor (smokers) at the top of the lungs but these cases are rarer. Working on posture, shoulder positioning, and relaxing the scalene and/or pec minor muscles can help. A pin and stretch or RI/PIR can be useful.

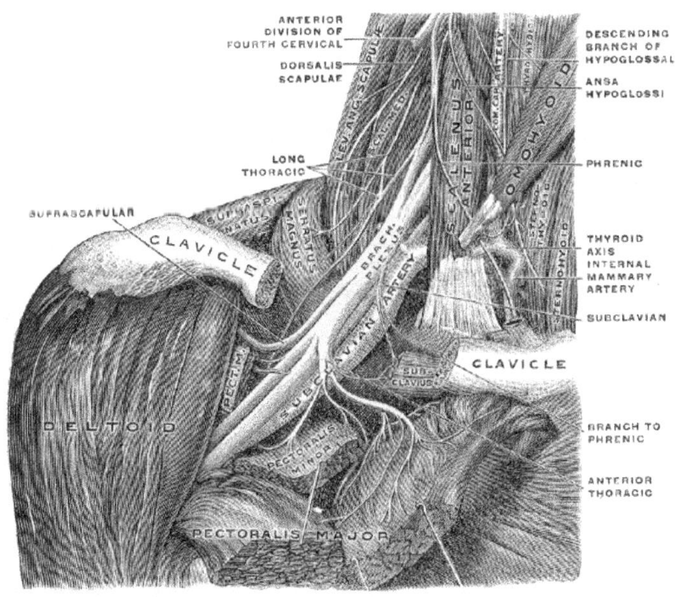

Shoulder impingement results in a sharp pain with lifting the arm right at the joint. The supraspinatus tendon and a bursa (cushion between the tendon and bone) both get pinched between the joint and the overhanging bone (acromion). This can be from poor muscle coordination, and the action being painful can be more protective, rather than from it causing damage. That being said, the pain could be damage or deconditioning related. There could be a tear and/or tendinosis of the supraspinatus tendon. There could be extra fluid in the bursa, limiting space. A musculoskeletal ultrasound or MRI may be handy for figuring out exactly what is going on. The solution for almost all problems is the same, though. Unless it is a large tear or full rupture, the solution in almost all cases is rehab. If there is damage or degenerative changes, rehab might take longer.

When is surgery indicated?

When the tear is large, the tendon is fully ruptured/torn, and/or there is a bone spur digging into the tendon then a surgical consult is recommended. Surgical outcomes are quite positive.[163]

When are injections indicated?

Injections are indicated if pain is too intense to start the exercises and/or if there is a lot of fluid in the bursa. Don't let someone inject steroids/cortisone into the tendon.

---

[163] Narvani AA, Imam MA, Godenèche A, Calvo E, Corbett S, Wallace AL, et al.Degenerative rotator cuff tear, repair or not repair? A review of current evidence. Ann R Coll Surg Engl. 2020; 102: 248-255
https://doi.org/10.1308/rcsann.2019.0173

What about frozen shoulder?

Frozen shoulder is also called adhesive capsulitis. A particular ligament (coracohumeral ligament) tightens which does not allow the shoulder to externally rotate. They physically are not capable, and the pain is extreme. Interestingly, this overdevelopment of the ligament is from an imbalance of the chemical messengers of the body that regulate ligament building and breakdown which causes the ligament to get bigger. It is very common for those with frozen shoulder to develop nodules/contractures at other locations, particularly in their palms. Those with diabetes are also at a higher risk. What I've described is true "frozen shoulder." Surgical release of the ligament, aggressive mobilizations to the ligament, and cortisone injections to the ligament are all effective treatments. Some doctors just inject the shoulder joint. Some target the coracohumeral ligament as much as possible with ultrasound imaging guidance.[164] I would get the ultrasound guided injection to the ligament to make sure the cortisone gets where it needs to be, as I want them to use the least amount to spare the joint as much as possible. Cortisone is destructive but, in this case, that is good since it can break down the ligament. Some people do get better with time, but others require soft tissue work and then some do require a medical intervention. Recovery time for frozen shoulder is normally 6 months to 2 years.

---

[164] McKean D, Chung SL, Naudé RTW, et al. Elasticity of the coracohumeral ligament in patients with frozen shoulder following rotator interval injection: a case series. *J Ultrason*. 2021;20(83):e300-e306. doi:10.15557/JoU.2020.0052

Post-injury or post-surgery, there might be muscle knots, muscle spasms, muscle shortening, or scar tissue, which can be painful and can limit some motions of the shoulder, and sometimes this is also called frozen shoulder. This type of frozen shoulder can normally be resolved much faster. I had patients come in with "frozen shoulder" that she had for 2 years since a car accident. I found a couple of painful muscle knots, so I treated them with ischemic compression. She left my office that day feeling 100% with full mobility.

Myofascial trigger points!

Those nasty muscle knots are **responsible for many chronic shoulder pains**. With almost any injury, the muscles will spasm to protect the shoulder. The overuse of the muscles will create muscle knots, and they can persist after the initial injury has healed. Also, they can be formed from pushing the body too hard (in terms of endurance): cooking in a restaurant, or doing yard work for 8 hours straight, etc. Counterintuitively, many muscle knots refer pain to other areas of the shoulder and sometimes down to the hand. The motion that creates the pain can give you a hint as to where the muscle knot may be. External rotation suggests infraspinatus/teres minor. Internal rotation suggests subscapularis. Lifting the arm suggests infraspinatus/teres minor and/or supraspinatus. The deltoid muscle does multiple motions. It tends to get achy, and if it is causing the pain, massaging it can help. See if the deltoid is tender, particularly near its distal attachment.

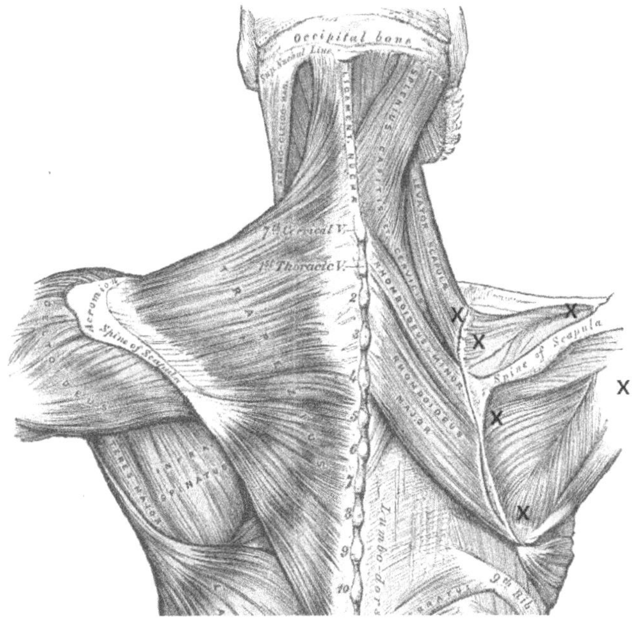

Common Shoulder Pain Muscle Knots 2

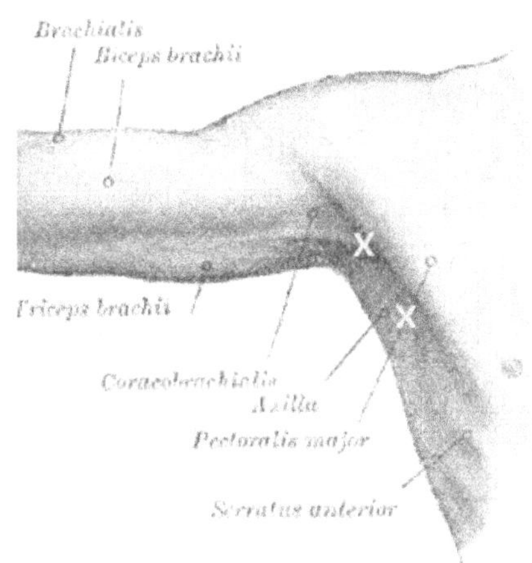

Tendinosis!

Tendinosis is a sickly tendon that is painful to use. The body hasn't been keeping up with the maintenance of the tendon, likely from lack of use. If you haven't exposed the tendon to large loads then the body might think it doesn't need to maintain that tendon. The wear and tear could also be a bit too much because the repair can't keep up properly, so poor shoulder coordination causing impingement can contribute. The best way to confirm a tendinosis is via musculoskeletal ultrasound imaging. The most typical tendon involved is the supraspinatus which is mostly responsible for lifting your arm upwards and over your head at your side. Lifting weights, improving muscle coordination to eliminate the impingement, light therapy, PRP, prolotherapy (dextrose), acupuncture, and fenestration may all be useful. Cortisone is not recommended unless absolutely necessary. If it is tendinosis and not a tear, then you can safely do the exercises even if they cause a bit of pain, maybe up to a 3/10 on the pain scale.

Recurring shoulder dislocations?

After an initial bad injury that dislocates the shoulder, the cup that holds the ball joint in place can become damaged, resulting in the shoulder being unstable and dislocating frequently. The cup is made of two parts: the bone and a cartilaginous and flexible rim called the labrum (the hip also has a labrum). Either one can be damaged (most common damage is called a Bankart lesion). If dislocation happen rarely enough, this might not be an issue, but if this is a chronic problem, then it can be resolved with surgery. They can repair the bony cup or anchor down the cartilaginous labrum.

The acromioclavicular (AC) joint

This joint is where the clavicle (collar bone) meets up with the acromion (the bony prominence just above the shoulder ball joint). This joint is one of the first joints in the body to start wearing out. By 40, most people have osteoarthritis in this joint. This is a good case to prove that arthritis doesn't equal pain because this joint rarely causes problems/pain in individuals and how bad it looks on X-ray or ultrasound rarely correlates to symptoms.[165] I have run into people with chronically tender AC joints, and the issue seems to resolve if all the shoulder and scapular (shoulder blade) muscles are working well together. Stretching tight muscles, mobilizing the joint, and exercises seems to help. Red light therapy has also seemed to help my patients if it is particularly tender (placebo effect?).

How to rehab the shoulder?

Shoulder rehab is very similar to neck or low back rehab. They are similar in that the joints have so many ways they can move and the joints involve so many muscles. Shoulder rehab has mostly two purposes: increase strength in any muscles that have atrophied and improve muscle coordination. For shoulders, unless a particular muscle is much worse than the others, I focus on control more than anything else. You can't just do one exercise. If your body masters just that one exercise, as soon as you try to move your shoulder in any other way, the joint will crack/pop, you'll get a jolt of pain, your muscles will spasm, and/or you'll be moving your shoulder blades instead of your arm. Variety is

---

[165] Rossano A, Manohar N, Veenendaal WJ, van den Bekerom MPJ, Ring D, Fatehi A. Prevalence of acromioclavicular joint osteoarthritis in people not seeking care: A systematic review. *J Orthop.* 2022;32:85-91. Published 2022 May 20. doi:10.1016/j.jor.2022.05.009

king. Slow and steady is king. If a motion is jittery, that motion is a perfect exercise to do daily until it is smooth (10-20 reps, 1-2 sets, 1-3x/day). Sometimes exercising in a mirror is important to check to see if your arm is doing what you ask it to. Check to see if your motions are symmetric. I recommend some weights or using exercise bands, but the amount of weight does not have to be much. Water bottles or soup cans can suffice. Of course, if you are shaking without weights, you don't need to add weights to that exercise. A typical exercise to do when you can't even lift the shoulder because of the impingement is arm swings and/or lifting the arm passively. So, if you have pinching pain with lifting the arm, you have to get your body used to moving your arm in that range. You can bend at the hip and let your arm hang, letting gravity "raise" your arm up for you. Another similar mobilization is using a broom handle to raise up your bad arm. Have the hand from your bad shoulder hold the handle and then use the good arm further down the broom to lift the bad arm without using any of the bad arm's muscles. You could also walk your hand up a wall. You could also put your hand onto a table or shelf and then move your body (bending over and/or sideways) to effectively "lift" the arm. If you are doing lots of exercises, particularly with weights, you can give yourself rest days, but to maximize efficiency in recovery, you can do very light shoulder motions on your rest days too.

Calcific Tendinitis

Calcific tendinitis is when the body starts to deposit calcium crystals into the tendon.[166] This can be quite painful but thankfully resolves well and relatively quickly in most. It can be more chronic and recurring in those with endocrine/hormone disorders, diabetes, or gout. Diagnosis can be confirmed with almost any form of medical imaging.

The crystals can be very chemically irritating, causing local inflammation. While not necessary for healing, cortisone injections into the bursa and nearby tissues (not into the tendon!) can help mitigate the pain. The crystals form a slurry and can normally be removed with a thick needle and this is considered the most effective treatment. Therapeutic ultrasound and extra corporeal shockwave therapy (ESWT) both seem to be effective at improving recovery, sometimes as effective as surgery. If recovery has stalled and you have tried for more than 6 months, then surgery can be considered. Keep in mind that maybe the initial calcific tendinitis has resolved and now the pain and limited range of motion might be from muscle knots, atrophy, muscle/ligament shortening, poor muscle coordination, etc.

---

[166] Kim MS, Kim IW, Lee S, Shin SJ. Diagnosis and treatment of calcific tendinitis of the shoulder. *Clin Shoulder Elb.* 2020;23(4):210-216. Published 2020 Nov 27. doi:10.5397/cise.2020.00318

ELBOW

The elbow has many muscles that cross it and a rather complicated and unique set of joints, but despite its complexity, there is little variety in the chronic problems found in this region.

The muscles that extend your fingers and wrist attach to the outside body prominence (lateral epicondyle) through a common tendon, and the muscles that flex your fingers and wrist attach to the inside bony prominence (medial epicondyle). Pain at the outside of the elbow is typically called lateral epicondylitis, or tennis elbow, and pain at the inside of the elbow is called medial epicondylitis, or golfer's elbow. These names are not that informative, though. They do communicate the typical aggravating activity, but "epicondylitis" is not really a thing. "Itis" implies inflammation and the epicondyle is the bony prominence. The pain there can be an angry bursa (bursitis), a ligament tear (sprain), a tendon tear, a tendinosis, or nearby muscle knots, but it isn't bone inflammation. In the more chronic scenario, it is likely to be muscle knots and/or tendinosis. A musculoskeletal ultrasound and a thorough check of the muscles attached to the tendons here can confirm the structure(s) causing the pain. Ischemic compression or dry needling could be used on the muscle knots, and the typical strategies for tendinosis can be used on the tendon: red light, eccentric exercises, PRP/prolotherapy injections, fenestration, acupuncture, etc. combined with a reduction or temporary avoidance of the aggravating activity such as golf or tennis.

Pronator Teres Syndrome

There are basically three nerves that cross the elbow (median, radial, and ulnar). The median nerve can be pinched just a couple inches distal and in front of the elbow. The muscle that can compress the nerve is called the pronator teres. This muscle might be tight (it typically is in most computer users) and/or it might have a muscle knot in it. The median nerve is responsible for grip strength and sensation for the front of the thumb, index, and middle finger, so weakness, tingling, or numbness there can be explained as coming from this muscular compression. It is always possible for nerves to be compressed in multiple locations, though, so keep an open mind. Muscle knots in the pronator teres tend to refer pain to the hand, mimicking nerve symptoms. Eliminating muscle knots in this muscle, stretching it, and keeping it relaxed might completely eliminate symptoms. This

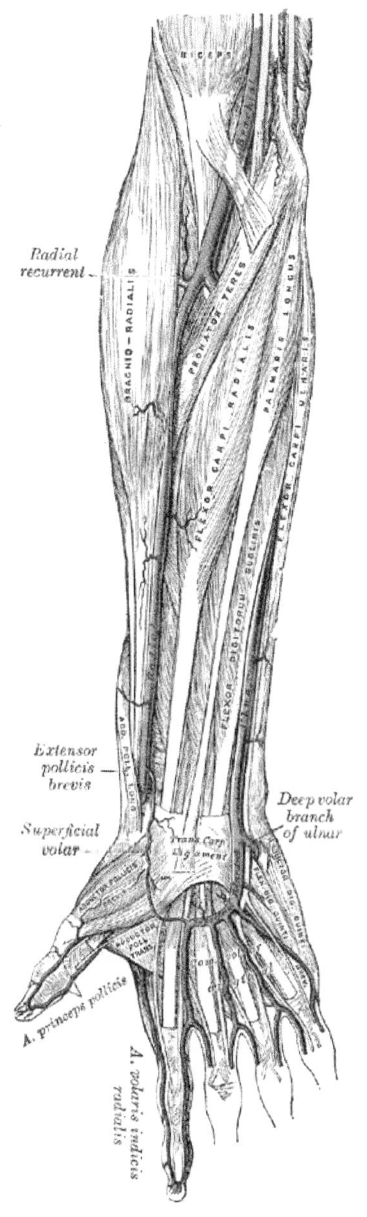

muscle is responsible for turning our hands downwards (like when we are typing). Sometimes this muscle can tighten every day, and I have shown office workers how to self-stretch this muscle to keep symptoms from coming back. Twenty seconds spent stretching at lunchtime every-day might be all that is necessary. I'll briefly describe it here.

If you place the palm of your opposite hand on the bone on the inside of the elbow then lie your thumb on your arm aiming towards the far side of the forearm, your thumb should be pointing along the pronator teres muscle. The idea is we will push on the muscle while it is relaxed and then lengthen the muscle while we are pushing on it, caus-ing a targeted stretch, then repeating until the muscle is re-laxed. (This is called a "pin-and-stretch"). It sometimes helps if the arm is relaxed sitting on your lap or on an arm-rest. Flop your arm so that the palm is downward. Then pin the muscle and flop your arm so the palm is upwards. If the thumb is in the right place and the muscle is tight you should be experiencing an achy/intense stretch. Hold for 3-6 seconds, then repeat the process. Sharp and/or spreading pain may be a muscle knot and ischemic compression should be used instead.

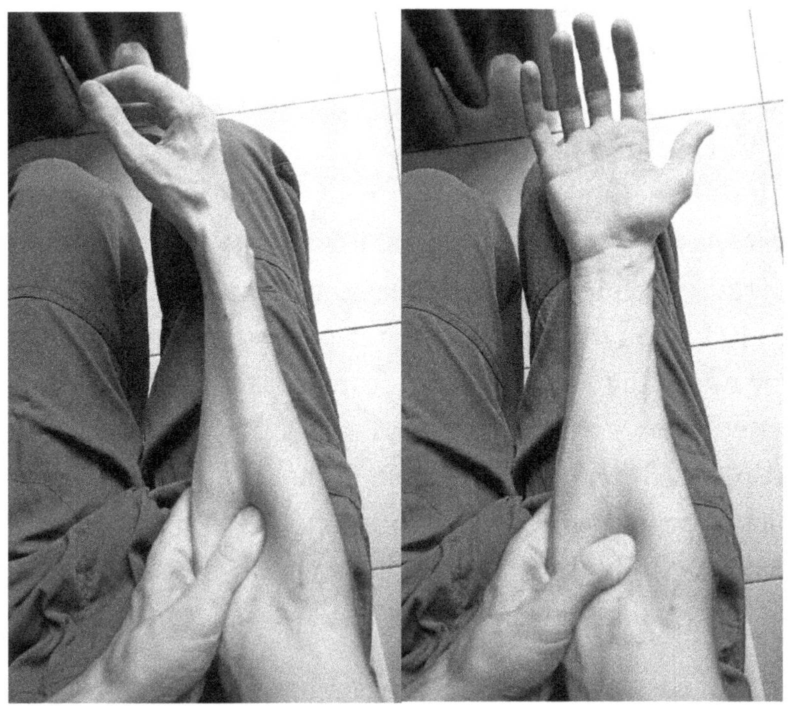

"Funny bone?"

The ulnar nerve runs behind the elbow along the inside of the arm and travels to the two smallest fingers. This is the "funny bone" location as the nerve is right between the skin and the bone here, so if it gets hit, the nerve pain can shoot down the arm. In terms of chronic issues, although much rarer compared to issues with the median nerve, the ulnar nerve can be compressed by tight muscles just an inch or two distal to the funny bone location. Another problem involving the ulnar nerve is that the nerve could also roll out of its groove as you flex the elbow. When the nerve snaps out of the groove, this can irritate it. Muscle work (exercises and massage/stretching) can resolve both issues, but there is a surgical option if non-surgical means don't work.

Elbow popping/clicking?

There is a particularly unique joint near the outside of the elbow. Our forearm is made of two long bones: the ulna and radius. The ulna stays still, but the radius can rotate and twist over the ulna (think hands down versus hands up). The radial head, the end of the radius which articulates with the elbow, is a round circle which is consistent with how the bone needs to move. This joint can be a source of discomfort particularly as someone extends the elbow. It can feel stuck, feel blocked, or can pop/click. Sometimes having a chiropractor or physiotherapist manipulate and mobilize this joint can eliminate or reduce this issue.

HAND/WRIST

We use our hands for so much that they are prone to injuries and a lot of wear and tear. In old age, the typical chronic problem is arthritis: the bony bumps, the spurs, and the joints don't run as well as they used to. Treatment for arthritis can help such as red-light therapy, diet/supplements, exercise, etc. Muscle knots in the forearm or shoulder can send pain to the hand and can be treated via dry needling and/or ischemic compression. Most hand muscles are in the forearm, but some pain can come from the muscles in the hand as well. Scar tissue from all the sprains and strains of the fingers can sometimes be a source of issues, and a thorough working out of the tissues can break up this scar tissue. Nerve compression/irritation at the neck, shoulder, forearm, and/or wrist can cause hand weakness, numbness, and/or pain.

Limited mobility/pinching

There are 8 tiny bones inside the wrist. The wrist can be one of those miracle chiropractic visits where I shake the joints of the wrist and they settle into a more comfortable location and the patient's "pinch" in their wrist is gone. A chiropractor or a physiotherapist should both be able to assess for limited mobility of these joints.

Trigger finger

Most muscles that control the fingers are in our forearms and not in our hands. The force gets transferred to the hand via tendons. To keep the tendons next to the bones, the tendons are held down with pulleys. A nodular tendon may no longer fit under the thickened pulley, either completely blocking the motion or resulting in a quick motion once the tendon finally pulls free. This is one of the cases where cortisone is the right choice as cortisone is destructive and can break down the tissue, allowing the tendon to fit under the pulley again.

Carpal tunnel syndrome (hand pain/weakness/numbness)

An overused diagnosis associated with an overdone surgical procedure with a poor success rate—not that some people don't have true carpal tunnel syndrome and not that surgery isn't an effective cure for some individuals. Carpal tunnel syndrome is diagnosed via hand nerve symptoms: pain, numbness, tingling, and weakness. In particular, weakness in grip and tingling/numbness in the fronts of the thumb, index, and middle finger. Hint: if you have nerve symptoms starting above the wrist, it isn't likely to be carpal tunnel (or just carpal tunnel). The median nerve, the nerve that innervates the skin of the thumb and first two fingers, passes in roughly the middle front of the wrist with all the tendons that flex the fingers. There is a ligamentous arch that keeps everything within the wrist called the flexor retinaculum. The theory is that the nerve is being compressed within the carpal tunnel, under the retinaculum, and the surgery is to cut this retinaculum, hoping to give the nerve some space. This is a very easy and quick surgery to do, and is really the only surgery done (outside of removing extra ribs) for nerve compression affecting the arm/hand, BUT... the wrist isn't the only place nerves can be compressed. The surgeon wants to help, so he does the only surgery he can do because he can't readily help if the nerve is compressed in a different location. This surgery is often advertised as having over a 90% success rate, but how is the success rate measured? If the symptoms improve at all, even temporarily, they can call it successful. The relief from surgery can be temporary and/or minor, so the patient goes on with their life thinking they will always have "carpal tunnel syndrome," and I don't call that a success. (I don't want to be too anti-surgery here—there are lots of people who do benefit from the surgery). With the increasing use of ultrasound imaging for nerve and muscle problems and the increasing availability as handheld ultrasound units become cheaper and more common, you should be able to find someone to get an image of the median nerve at the wrist. They can easily see if the wrist is likely causing the nerve compression. I've been starting every "carpal tunnel" case by looking at the nerve at the wrist, and it has only been compressed there maybe 20-30% of the time.

Everyone is allowed to have more than one problem. Even if you do have carpal tunnel syndrome, maybe the nerve is also compressed at the forearm, the shoulder, or the neck. Maybe there are muscle knot pains. Maybe you don't have carpal tunnel at all and it is just muscle pains and/or from the neck. Maybe it is a vitamin B12 deficiency or diabetes, which can both cause nerve symptoms. It could be a random mix of problems to create your unique combination. In my experience (working in the Cayman Islands with lots of lawyers and accountants), the forearm is the most common nerve impingement site. This problem doesn't require surgery and is easily resolved, often in one visit. It is called pronator teres syndrome, and is discussed in the elbow section. For the other nerve impingement sites, see the shoulder (TOS) and neck (radiculopathy) sections.

BACK/PELVIS

There are normally only 4 pain generators in the back and pelvis: the muscles, the facet joints, the discs, and the sacro-iliac joints. Nerve pain in the back is rarer, as when nerves are involved the nerve symptoms tend to be in the legs. People underestimate how high the pelvis is, as many people's "low back pain" is from the pelvis or from the pelvis muscles. Many people's "sciatica" pain down the back of their legs with their "low back pain" is muscle knots in the gluteal region referring pain down the leg. Back problems are similar to neck problems in terms of causes and solutions, and pelvis problems can also be hip problems, so it may be useful to read the neck and hip sections as well.

Can you tell what structure is causing the pain?

Sometimes you can. Often it is a mix of multiple issues which muddies the water. Pain can travel and/or central sensitization may create pain not related to any damage. What movements aggravate the pain and where the pain is can help focus diagnosis and treatment to certain structures/regions. One way to find painful structures is to carefully inject an anesthetic in one specific location, and if there is pain relief there, we can localize the pain as coming from that region (a very important step if surgery/nerve ablation is being considered for pain).

Back muscle pain tends to be localized to the region. Pelvis/hip muscle pain tends to refer across the base of the sacrum/pelvis, deep into the hip joint, and/or down the leg.

A painful disc hates sitting and bending forward the most. Bearing down, like using the toilet or blowing out candles, can aggravate disc pain. Surprisingly, they normally tolerate standing and walking well and people can get relief after bending backwards (repeated or sustained holds) as most injured discs actually like bending backwards. Most disc issues happen in people's 30s and 40s and are rare in the elderly. Even if you had a disc issue in the past, your recurrent back pain might not be the disc anymore.

The facet joints hate bending backwards, and this motion can aggravate the sacroiliac (SI) joints too. The facet joints also dislike standing/walking. They feel better sitting and bending forward. Facet joint pain prevalence increases with age, so this is more likely to be a contributor to chronic pain in the elderly.

SI joints hate moving. The act of getting up would be more painful than either sitting or standing. Standing might be fine, but walking might hurt. Pain is normally sharp and located mostly at one of the two bony protrusions: the PSISs. If someone comes in and they say they get sharp pain and they point with a single finger right to a PSIS, it is called Fortin's finger sign and is a strong indication that the SI joint is causing some, if not all, of the pain. There are muscle knots just outside the PSIS in the glutes that can mimic SI problems or may be bothering the patient concurrently.

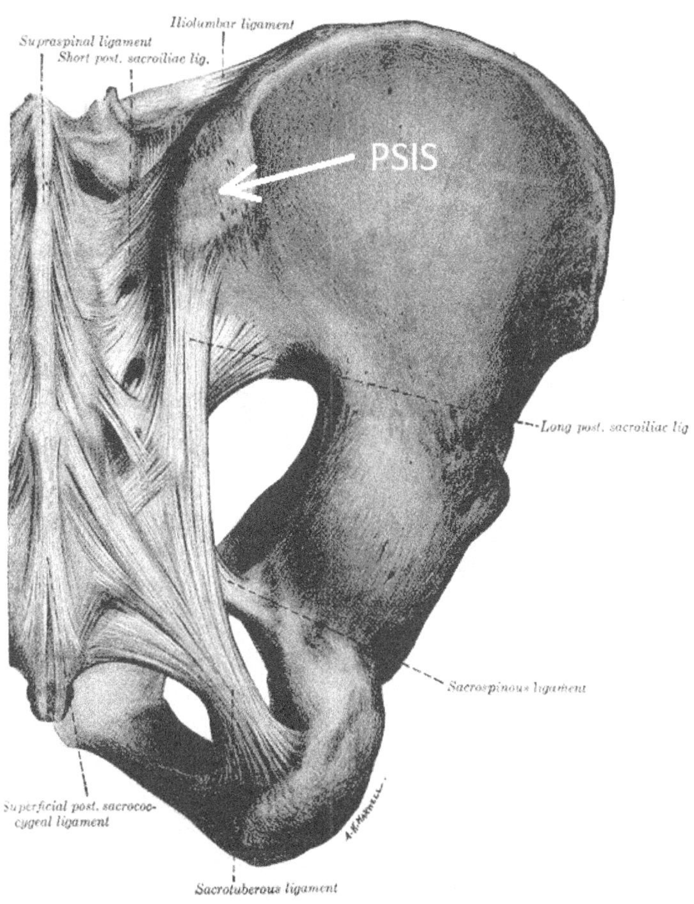

"But I had an imaging done, and they said I had..."

I've said it before and I'll say it again: pain ≠ damage. Degenerative changes in the spine are common and don't necessarily cause any pain. You could argue lots of chiropractors and medical doctors are responsible for chronic pain syndromes and central sensitization as they point to an image and say, "There is your problem! This structure is broken, your back is no good anymore!" The negative imagery presented to your subconscious mind can lead to protective muscles spasms, pain to keep you from moving, and increased pain sensitivity. There is a nearby chart I've provided of imaging findings in asymptomatic individuals. This gives you an idea for how normal some of these findings are. One third to one half of people with no back pain have a disc protrusion (a disc herniation) when imaged! So, if you go to a doctor and get an MRI and they say, "AHA, disc problem!" Is it really the disc? My radiograph instructors would always remind us to treat the patient, not the image. I'll also remind you again of the saying, "A picture of a telephone doesn't tell you if it is ringing."

Systematic Literature Review of Imaging Features of Spinal Degeneration in Asymptomatic Populations (pain-free individuals)[167] (W. Brinkikji *et. al.* 2015)							
	Age (yr)						
Imaging findings	**20**	**30**	**40**	**50**	**60**	**70**	**80**
Disc degeneration	37%	52%	68%	80%	88%	93%	96%
Disc signal loss	17%	33%	54%	73%	86%	94%	97%
Disc height loss	24%	34%	45%	56%	67%	76%	84%
Disc Bulge	30%	40%	50%	60%	69%	77%	84%
Disc Protrusion	29%	31%	33%	36%	38%	40%	43%
Annular fissure	19%	20%	22%	23%	25%	27%	29%
Facet Degeneration	4%	9%	18%	32%	50%	69%	83%
Spondylolisthesis	3%	5%	8%	14%	23%	35%	50%

---

[167] Brinjikji W, Luetmer PH, Comstock B, et al. Systematic literature review of imaging features of spinal degeneration in asymptomatic populations. *AJNR Am J Neuroradiol.* 2015;36(4):811-816. doi:10.3174/ajnr.A4173

Do you have chronically tight and achy back muscles?

With almost any back injury or back pain the longer muscles of the back will kick in and splint the back to add stability and to protect it. In fact, a lot of acute locked backs start with sharp pain from the joints or a disc, but shift to pain from the long muscles being so tired and achy from working all-day, every-day, since the pain started. In chronic cases, your back can be tight continuously as your brain doesn't trust that the back is good/safe, so remains permanently in protection mode. This mode is often most intense upon first getting up in the morning as you have to convince your brain to let you start moving your back at all. If this has persisted for a while, you may be experiencing central sensitization where pain sensitivity is ramped up and moving might be painful as part of the body's protection system. As an advocate and user of ultrasound imaging, I have an interest in current research, and there are researchers toying with the idea of measuring muscle sizes in the back to determine how chronic/bad someone's back is. They look at the ratio between the long/splinting muscles (quadratus lumborum - QL) and the tiny fine-motor control muscles (multifidus). If your back has been moving stiffly for years, your brain might have forgotten how to use the fine motor muscles, and they end up wasting away (atrophied). While the exact ratio is still up for debate, when it is really off, their ability to predict chronic back tightness and/or back lock-ing/spasms is basically perfect.[168]

There are some simple ways of relaxing the muscles, but the muscle tightness may return if the body is used to, and re-lies on, keeping those muscles tight. **You need back re-training to get the fine motor muscles working again before the long muscles will stay relaxed**. If the problem is not that chronic, then relaxing the muscles may provide sufficient relief that you may be one of those people that gets "maintenance" type care by a physio/chiro/massage therapist.

How to relax the low back muscles?

Massage and/or heat might help. Joint mobilization/chiro-practic adjustments might help. In my experience, dry nee-dling/acupuncture, pin-and-stretch, and muscle energy techniques are the most effective at relaxing the back mus-cles (relief may be temporary). Pin-and-stretch and muscle energy techniques are simple enough you could do them at home with a partner (or go to see your physio/chiro). I'll describe the pin-and-stretch here.

---

[168] Huang Q, Zhang Y, Li D, Yang D, Huo M, Maruyama H. The Evaluation of Chronic Low Back Pain by Determining the Ratio of the Lumbar Multifidus Muscle Cross-sectional Areas of the Unaffected and Affected Sides. *J Phys Ther Sci.* 2014;26(10):1613-1614. doi:10.1589/jpts.26.1613

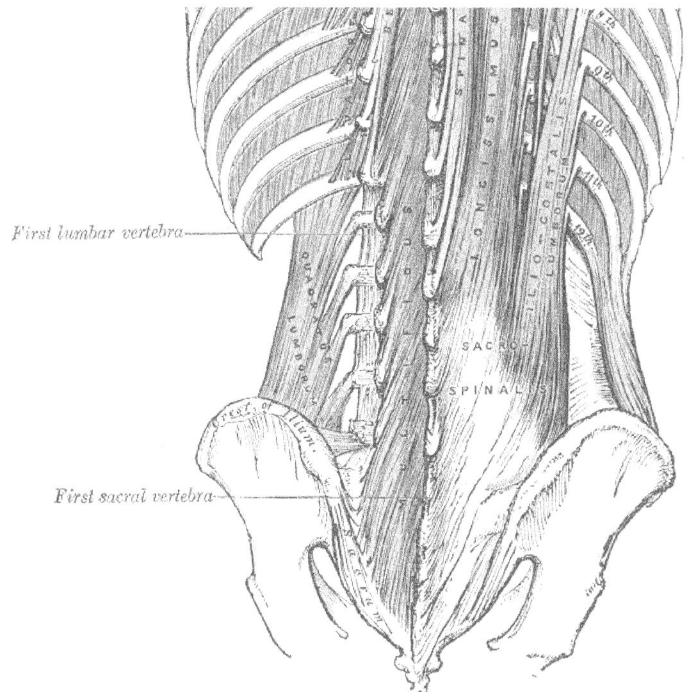

First, I have the person sit on a bench, stool, or sideways on a chair. The important part is that I have access to their back and they can bend forward and sideways. I push on the quadratus lumborum (QL), which will be the tight/tender steel cables connecting the ribs to the pelvis that will be palpable as you go from their flanks towards the spine. Once I have firm pressure there, the patient slowly bends diagonally forward, away from the contact point, to stretch it. If done well the patient will feel an intense achy stretch. Repeat, slightly moving the pressure point each time, until tenderness and tightness are reduced. This can be repeated for the muscles of the low back along the spine by bending forwards instead of diagonally, but those are definitely so strong you can't use fingers and must use something firm like a trigger point tool, the handle of a screwdriver, etc.

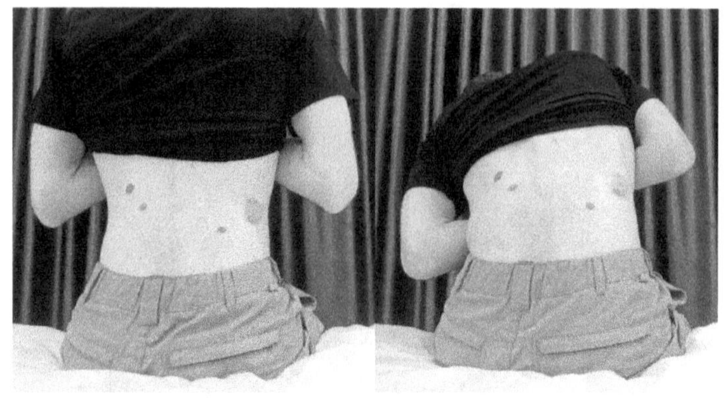

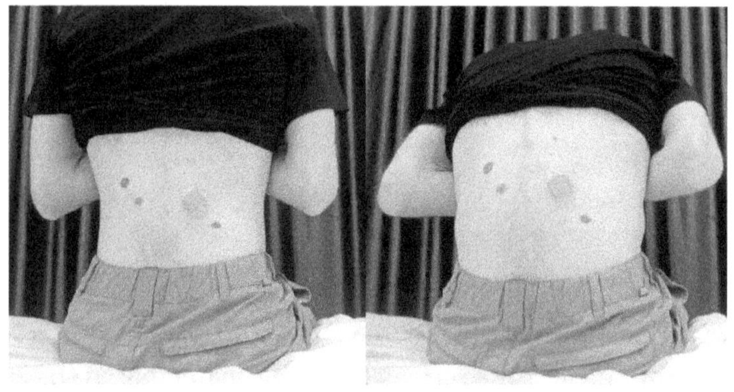

Does your back "go out" or "lock up" if you aren't careful?

This is, of course, linked to the chronic tightness in the low back. The fine motor control muscles of the back are atrophied from years of you moving stiffly. Your body has forgotten all about those muscles. Now if you bend forward and try to come back up, the control can mess up causing the joints to buckle and temporarily move improperly. This may result in a minor sprain and/or joint pinch. The damage can be negligible, but whether there is a minor injury/inflammatory response or not, the body's response is not negligible. The body locks down everything with muscle spasms, and it makes moving painful to lock you in place. Something just moved wrong, and it is scared it may happen again if it lets you continue to move. While chiropractic, acupuncture, physio, heat/cold, TENS, and/or time can help you recover from that incident, every incident results in more of the chronic tightness/achiness in the back and more fear of moving. The long-term solution is to retrain and recondition the back.

There is a second type of back "going out" involving the pelvis/SI joints instead of the lumbar (lower) spine to consider, which may require combined hip and back related treatments/rehab. The SI joint being "out of place" in particular can respond well to chiropractic adjustments with immediate relief. Even if you get relief, if the problem is chronic, rehab may be necessary to keep it from coming back.

What about a back brace?

The short answer is… no. All types of braces may be needed in acute injuries and there can be usefulness in having a pelvic/SI belt… but a back brace for the lumbar spine will never be recommended by a physio therapist or a chiropractor. Well… if you won't do exercises and you are getting some relief from it, they might feel defeated enough to not stop you from using it. The brace will further weaken the control muscles and you will become reliant on it. You become scared to move without it. It is not a good long-term solution.

A weightlifting belt is similar to a back brace for professional weightlifting where they are pushing their bodies to the limits and they can benefit from extra support to prevent injury. Lumbar supports in seats are useful and are recommended.

Sacroiliac (SI) Joint Pain

As mentioned before, this is a sharp pain, normally aggravated by movements. If you point right to the pelvis bony prominence (PSIS) with one finger, then chances are this is contributing or causing your pain.

The pelvis is made of 3 bones: the sacrum which is a triangular shaped bone connecting to the spine above it and having the tailbone (coccyx) at its other end, and the ilia (the wings). The joint between the sacrum and the ilia could be the issue. This joint only has a few degrees of motion, but you could imagine if it is sitting at, or moved to, the extremes of its range, this can result in a sharp pinch, pressure, and/or a crooked/twisted feeling in the pelvis. Sometimes the issue is described as an instability, being misaligned, or being out-of-place.

This joint is unique in many ways, and one such way is that there are no muscles that directly strengthen the joint. No muscle goes from the ilia to the sacrum. There is no muscle to strengthen to stabilize and reinforce this joint. Muscles go from spine to the ilia/sacrum or from the sacrum/ilia to the leg. Stability comes from the ligaments/shape of the joint and from the coordination of the muscles from the back and hip. The SI joint can get all out of whack during pregnancy due to the hormone relaxin which loosens the ligaments to allow the pelvis to flex and move much more than normal, but SI issues can strike anyone. The issue may start with an injury to the pelvis where the ligaments become damaged. The lack of regular movement during healing can result in faulty muscle coordination patterns resulting in a less stable SI joint, resulting in recurring bouts of SI pain. Most typically, a bout of SI pain gets triggered by coming up from bending forward or twisting quickly.

So how is it treated? I would consider an SI issue to be one of the two issues most likely to be resolved (at least temporarily) with a chiropractic adjustment (The other being acute rib pain/pain with deep breaths). If we can get that pelvis sitting comfortably, the pain can go down to near zero in a single session. If it moved so far that a ligament was sprained, then it will require time for healing. I might recommend temporary, as required, use of a sacral belt, which squeezes the ilia together. You can check to see if this would benefit you by having someone squeeze your ilia together and then you would perform a movement that would normally be painful. If the pain is less, then look into purchasing/using a belt. Use it as little as possible though. DON'T become reliant on it. Excessive use can result in more joint instability. If this issue is more chronic, then muscle knots may also have to be treated, which may take more than one session. In fact, I think some people's muscle knot pain was hiding until nearby SI pain starts and then the brain is like, "Hey, while you're in the area, there's some other pain I've been ignoring I should tell you about." Often muscle work, combined with either quick thrusts or gentle pressure on the joint should be used. The gentle pressure style uses blocks called sacral or pelvic blocks. These wedges use your own body weight to try to coax the joint back into its comfy spot. In chronic cases, the problem might return unless low back and/or hip rehab is done.

Some practitioners are squeamish about working in the area of the pelvis. For example, the sacrotuberous ligament should be checked, but it is right next to the anus, so some chiros and physios don't check it. You may want a physio who specializes in pelvic work, and if you are a woman, you may want a female physio. One of my biggest criticisms of chiropractic is chiropractors who only do the joint manipulations/chiropractic adjustments. If you see a chiro who has done "Webster" training, they should be comfortable at least doing a little soft tissue treatment into the psoas, piriformis, and sacrotuberous ligaments.

Common Pelvis/Low-back Pain Muscle Knots

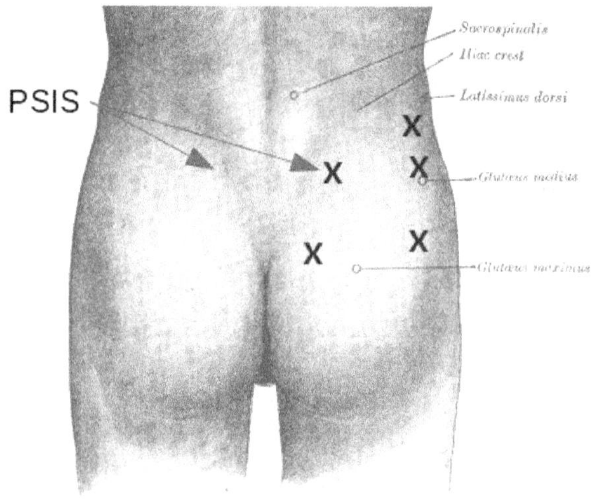

BRANDON RAMAKKO

Tailbone pain?

The coccyx (tailbone) and its joint with the sacrum can be a source of chronic pain. Some people have a big coccyx and some small (why does that sound lewd?). This is our vestigial tail. For some, the coccyx is solid bone and for others it is segmented. Often the joint between it and the sacrum gets a little uncomfortable or out of place. This can be from a fall or giving birth. Working on the muscles that attach to it or nearby can sometimes be enough to get things comfortable again. You want to find a practitioner comfortable working in the pelvis in proximity to the anus. Some practitioners, for stubborn cases of pelvic pain, work the pelvic muscles through the anus and/or vagina. In extreme cases, chiropractors can go through the anus to hook onto the front of the coccyx and try to pull it back where it should be. Due to the unconventional nature of the procedure, many states have this treatment explicitly written into the scope of practice for chiropractors because it is such a weird thing for a chiropractor to do. I don't know any chiropractor personally who has done it, and thankfully, all my coccyx pain patients have gotten better without requiring this treatment. In the event the pain is definitely coming from the coccyx, and it isn't getting better, they can surgically remove it and the results are pretty good.[169]

---

[169] Sagoo NS, Haider AS, Palmisciano P, et al. Coccygectomy for refractory coccygodynia: a systematic review and meta-analysis. *Eur Spine J.* 2022;31(1):176-189. doi:10.1007/s00586-021-07041-6

Maigne's syndrome (cluneal nerve neuropathy)

There is a superficial nerve called the cluneal nerve that runs from the spine starting at the bottom of the rib cage, then travels along the path of the QL, and then splits into three to travel onto the glutes, over the lateral hip, and one branch curving into the inguinal crease (front hip crease). This nerve can be responsible for burning, tingling, numbness, and/or electrical/shooting pain in these regions. This problem can be called Maigne's syndrome. I've had a 100% success rate at eliminating this, once identified, in a session or two. The nerve can get caught up in the fascia if there are fascial adhesions under the skin. It can also be bothered at the joint where it exits the spine (bottom of rib cage). In fact, many people describe/experience intense stiffness at the base of the rib cage, just beneath the bra strap for women.

Mobilizing the joints either gently, or with a chiropractic adjustment, is where I typically start. I then free up the skin along the path of the nerve using quick tissue thrusts or slide cupping in regions where the skin isn't gliding properly in all directions.

"What about my old disc herniation? My pain must be from that!"

Maybe... But unlikely. Let's delve into how discs work. The discs have gooey, fluid-filled centers and a ring of fibers going around the edge (the annulus). When pressure is applied to the disc, the gel/fluid wants to get squished outwards, and the annulus holds it in. The disk takes a compressive force and converts it into a tensile force with the annulus fibers in tension instead of compression. We have no pain receptors within the inner disc fibers, so they can get damaged without us knowing. This is why some people's disc pain starts when doing something trivial they've done 1000 times before. It was just that the damage finally extended to a nerve receptor in the outer third of the annulus. People can have disc bulges and herniations without pain, and people can have disc pain without a herniation.

Fresh disc herniations are the painful ones. In particular, if the gooey stuff leaks out. The body doesn't recognize the stuff and attacks it, causing a lot of local inflammation. The stuff could physically compress the nerve roots or the spinal cord, or the inflammation may irritate the nearby nerve roots. The short-term nerve pain can be due to this inflammatory effect. In the majority of cases, the stuff gets cleaned up and the disc pain resolves. In my clinical experience, most people's "sciatica" and "disc is out again" pain has nothing to do with the nerves or the discs. The "sciatica" is referred pain from muscle knots, and the disc pain has been replaced with the chronic tightness and segmental instability talked about earlier in this section. In particular, I notice they are scared of the motion that caused the first incident, and the muscle control is worse with that motion because they avoid it. If they do end up in that position, the joints buckle, causing protective pain and spasms from the uncoordinated movements/pinching. It is important to rehab and relearn the movements that they have been fearing in a safe and comfortable manner.

The elderly don't get fresh disc herniations anymore because the disc is dried out: there is nothing to be squirted out. The disc does heal with scar tissue (which isn't as strong as the original tissue) and the body does add in extra "pain" receptors deeper into the disc where there wasn't any before. The combination of both factors might lead to some disc-type pain even if, due to age, a big disc herniation is unlikely. Disc pain normally responds extremely well to repeated extreme backward bends or sustained back extension (the cobra yoga pose). Sometimes, sideways hip glides work better. This type of exercise is prescribed by any physiotherapist or chiropractor who knows what they are doing for disc pain. Caution though, as mentioned here, later in life the disc is much less likely to cause pain/problems, and these exercises can exacerbate other issues as these motions stress the facet joints and the SI joints, and if they are irritated already, they won't be happy. For disc pain aggravation, I normally recommend 10 repetitions every hour and walking as much as possible—as long as the activities are continuing to reduce pain and/or improve motion. If the exercises reduce leg pain but slightly increase back pain, that is still an indication to continue.

Nerve pinching

Nerve symptoms coming from the back could be due to chemical irritation of nerves, reduced blood flow to nerves, and/or compression of nerves. Severe or worsening nerve symptoms are reasons to get an MRI and back surgery.

The chemical irritation could be from an injury to nearby structures. This is painful, but doesn't normally result in loss of sensation or strength. Normally, the solution is to fix whatever else is going on, and the nerve issue will resolve itself.

Batson's venous plexus drains the blood away from the nerves, but if the blood flow is backed up, then the nerves will receive less fresh blood and nutrients. These malnourished nerves won't work as well, resulting in sensory loss and weakness (maybe pain, too). This is a less studied issue, mostly because it resolves easily. Getting the segments of the back moving freely can help the blood start flowing well again, and the issue can resolve.

Nerve compression can be from a tumor, from bone spurs on the joints (remember that arthritis isn't necessarily painful), from a recent or old disc herniation/bulge, from the spinal segments sliding too far, and/or from ligament thickening. If the compression is such that the muscle/limb barely moves when activated, that is a sign for urgent imaging and surgery. If the nerve symptoms involve bowel and urinary control or sexual function, that is an urgent/emergent condition.

A tumor/cancer is its own serious issue beyond the scope of this book. Gradually worsening symptoms can be a sign of a growing tumor. Many types of cancer spread to bone when they metastasize such as breast, lung, and prostate cancer. We will focus on worsening nerve symptoms with a structural cause in the next section, because it is often associated with instability and age.

Structural instability and chronic nerve symptoms

As we age, our discs bulge out a bit more, all of our spinal joints become spikier, the ligamentum flavum (ligament running down the back of the spinal canal) thickens and can bunch up when bending backwards or standing, and the L4 vertebrae starts to slide forward on L5. Eventually, everyone starts to get nerve symptoms from this, provided they live long enough. Also, L5 can slide forward on the sacrum (pelvis), but this tends to only happen to individuals who have broken their L5, and when the body repaired the fracture, the joints and the vertebral body remained separate so that they can grow further apart over time. Interestingly, most people who have this non-union fracture don't remember hurting their back as it tends to happen in the teen years in those who participated in contact sports or gymnastics/cheerleading. A standard MRI sometimes doesn't tell the whole story as in a standard MRI you are recumbent (lying on your back), but your symptoms might only be apparent when standing (particularly the sliding of the vertebra, called a structural instability). A standing MRI or MRI combined with X-ray may be required to get a picture of the structure/problem affecting the nerve. If nerve symptoms are worsening, or even persisting, then surgery is often the best recourse (assuming you tried the other things in this book). They can fuse the vertebrae together, getting rid of the sliding problem. This solution does require your other vertebra to do more work after surgery. They can shave off the bone spurs and trim off the disc bulge. Disc bulge/protrusion/herniation trimming is a fairly unobtrusive surgery nowadays. Look for those advertising a minimally invasive discectomy or an endoscopic/laparoscopic discectomy. Another possible surgery is removing part of the posterior arch of the vertebra to give the canal more room.

HIP

The hip joint works similarly to the shoulder joint. The anatomy is similar, and the problems are similar. It is a ball and socket joint. There is a soft cup called a labrum which helps hold the head in the joint. There are muscles, equivalent to the rotator cuff, which help control and move the joint. This joint is more prone to arthritis than the shoulder. It is similarly prone to tendon tears, tendinosis, and muscle knots causing pain. As written earlier in the book, arthritis isn't necessarily painful, and many individuals with pretty bad hip arthritis on X-ray have no hip problems/pain. The majority of chronic hip pains are from muscle and tendon problems. Back pain and nerve compression in the back/pelvis can refer to the hip, so be sure to read that section as well.

Burning thigh pain?

Burning nerve pain, tingling, and/or numbness along the anterolateral (front+outside) thigh can be from a superficial peripheral nerve that comes out just below and inside of the anterolateral bony protrusion of the pelvis (ASIS). This nerve is called the lateral femoral cutaneous nerve and innervates the skin in the region of the anterolateral thigh. The nerve can be pinched/irritated/entrapped where it comes out of the pelvis. This issue is sometimes called "meralgia paresthetica," a neuralgia, a neuropathy, or a peripheral nerve entrapment. I've had a surprisingly high success rate so far with pulling/shaking the nerve free. I have the patient lunge forward with the painful leg ending up behind them. As they move, I am imagining grabbing the nerve where it comes out of the pelvis with my thumb and I thrust/push/pull the tissue/muscles there, just below the bony prominence. If this doesn't resolve it, I check along the skin too. This nerve runs just under the skin, so I make sure the skin is gliding well. If it isn't, I use quick thrusts or slide cupping to free up the skin.

Just like any other nerve issue, a vitamin B12 deficiency or diabetes can cause it. In fact, this is one of the first nerve symptoms to appear with diabetes. If this is the case, this problem may only be treatable by treating the underlying issue.

"Trochanteric bursitis"

This is a mostly archaic diagnosis that is still sometimes being used. They scanned via MRI or ultrasound people with painful hips and saw fluid in the bursa near the greater trochanter (the outermost part of the hip where the gluteal tendons pass by or attach). They assumed the fluid was from some sort of inflammatory process so they labeled it an "itis". It was normally treated by injecting the bursa with cortisone. While some bursas are painful and inflamed, the hip bursa is not the source of pain unless it is infected (which is rare) even if there is fluid on imaging. They now know that if there is extra fluid in the bursa, it isn't the source of pain, but it is indicative that there is a problem with the nearby tendons: tendinosis and/or tendon tears. Of course, I still see patients who have been diagnosed with this without imaging, just based on the presence of hip pain, and in their cases, their pain could be muscle knots, tendon issues, cluneal nerve entrapment, or referred pain from the back/pelvis.

Muscle knots

Just like every section in this book, muscle knots can be a part of the chronic pain or the entire problem. They can refer the pain down the back of the leg, down the front/side of the leg, the inguinal crease (front crease), deep in the hip joint, and/or across the pelvis. They can mimic "sciatica." The muscles involved can be the tensor fascia latae (TFL), glutes, vastus lateralis, piriformis, iliacus, psoas, and more rarely, the hamstrings. It is very common, particularly for women, to develop hip pain as they age that becomes uncomfortable when they lie on their side. In particular, it tends to be muscle knots in the TFL. Once treated, these muscle knots might never return or take many months/years to return, but remember that muscle knots form when muscles are asked to stay active longer than is necessary. The muscle recruitment patterns of the hips can be messed up, and if it isn't fixed, then the muscle knots return. See the muscle knot locations in the nearby images and in the back section as well.

Common Hip/Leg Pain Muscle Knots 1

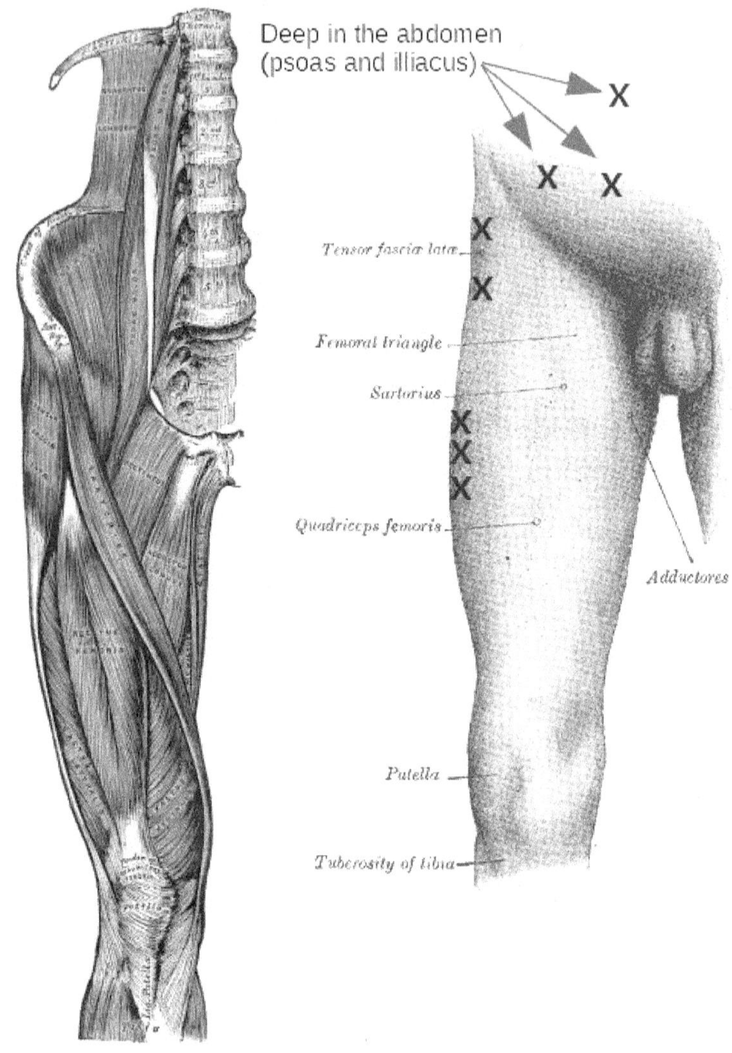

Common Hip/Leg Pain Muscle Knots 2

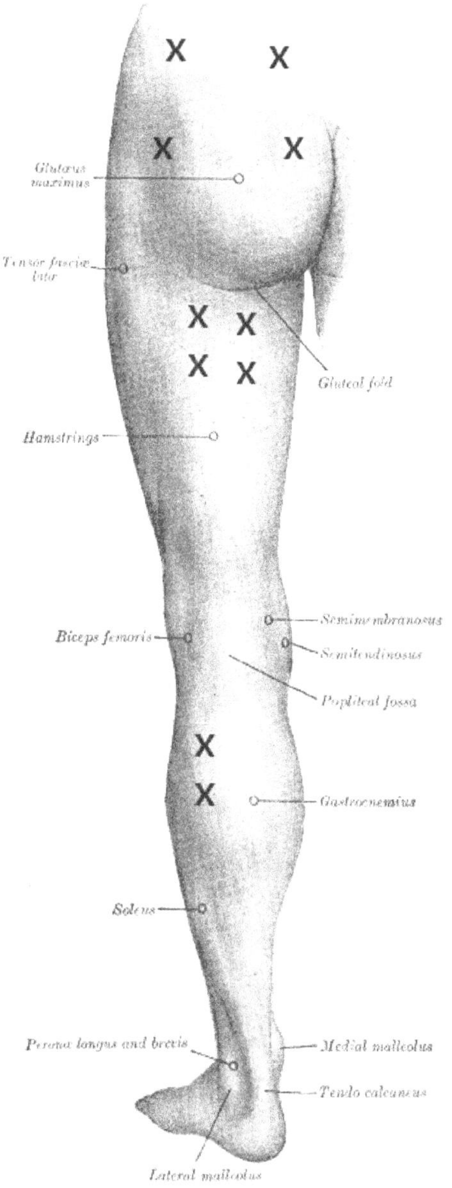

Piriformis syndrome

The piriformis muscle knots are known for referring down the leg. The sciatic nerve also goes down the back of the leg. If the only symptom is pain down the back of the leg starting in the hip region, it could be muscle knots in the piriformis, or the piriformis could be compressing the sciatic nerve. If there is muscle weakness or numbness, then the nerve is definitely involved. The solution is the same: treat the muscle knots in the piriformis and maybe stretch the piriformis, too. Remember that everyone is allowed to have as many problems as they want, and if you only get partial relief, then nerve compression might be in the spine/back and/or the pain might be from any of the other pelvis/hip muscles in the glute/hamstring area.

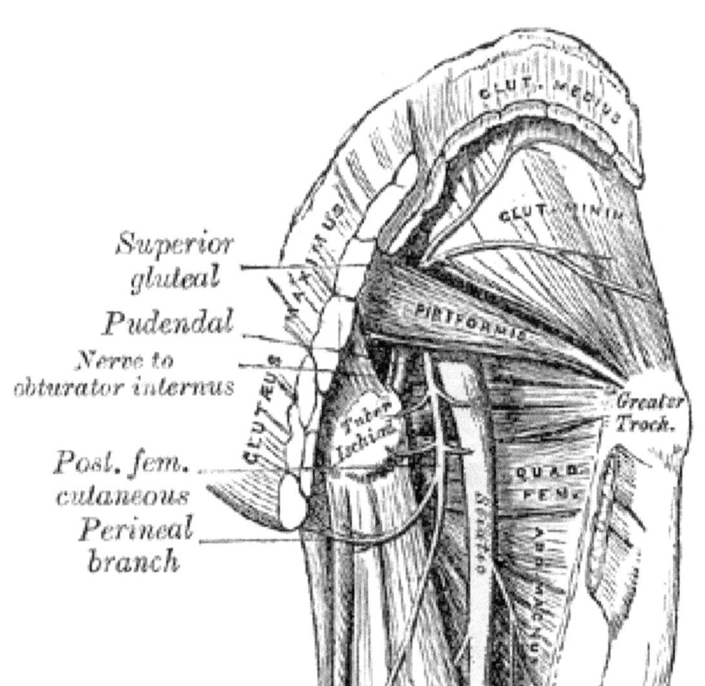

Chronically Tight IT Band

The tensor fascia latae (TFL) is a common muscle to over-work because it is a helper. It can do a little of everything: externally rotating the leg, lifting the hip, and bringing the leg forward. It is the main muscle that tenses the iliotibial band (IT band). All those times you are stretching the IT band, you are really stretching the TFL muscle (the IT band doesn't actually lengthen) and maybe massaging your vastus lateralis. The main muscle which is supposed to be lifting the hip is the gluteus medius (glute med). I often find this muscle atrophied if the problem of TFL overuse has persisted for years. There is a hollow where the muscle should be as the muscle has weakened/wasted away, but it can be bulked up again! If you can get this muscle to be active again, then the "chronic IT band tightness" can finally be resolved along with preventing the recurrence of painful muscle knots. This issue with the overworked TFL and weakened/deactivated glute med typically results in muscle knots in the TFL (check the gluteal region too) and vastus lateralis. This issue is often combined with clicking knees with squats and stairs (see the knee section). Targeted exercises and correcting bad walking and stair climbing habits can quickly strengthen the glute med muscle and improve its participation.

The exercise I often give people is "standing hip abduction." But I've seen plenty of YouTube videos and websites where the demonstrator is "cheating a bit," and I've seen physiotherapy assistants not know the difference between doing it "right" or "wrong." Before I continue, there is rarely a "wrong" way to do an exercise, just different ways for different purposes. In our case, we want to emphasize the glute med and de-emphasize the TFL which is going to try and take over the exercise if we let it.

Standing hip abduction is lifting your leg towards the side. An overactive TFL user is going to want to subconsciously use the TFL. The TFL wants to turn the toes outwards and wants the leg to go in a diagonal. Even if they try to bring the leg directly towards the side, they don't realize their pelvis will tilt forward effectively creating the same diagonal motion at the hip joint. So, stand straight, hold a bit of a hip thrust to keep from cheating at the pelvis, rotate the foot/leg inwards, and lift the leg directly towards the side. It doesn't have to go very high. If you have a hard time doing this exercise without cheating in some way, you really need this exercise.

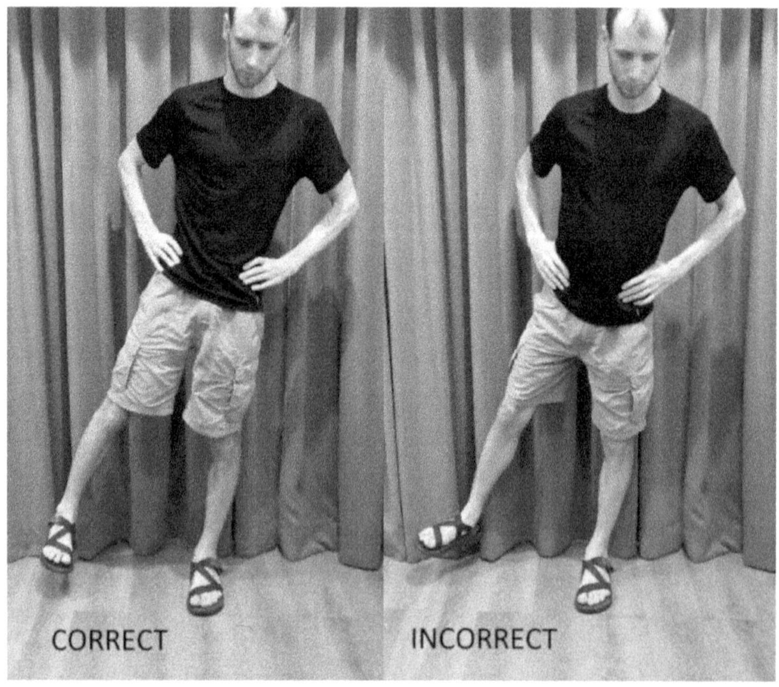

Extreme weakness and pain with lifting the hip

While some amount of glute med pain/dysfunction is typical with any hip/pelvis problem, we have to be on guard for extreme weakness and pain. Since glute med is the main hip lifter, if the patient is unable to keep their pelvis level while standing on one foot, then it may be possible that they have torn the glute med tendon or it is tearing, likely with tendinosis as well. This hip drop is called a Trendelenburg sign and called a Trendelenburg gait when it is noticed while they are walking. **A full tear can be repaired surgically, even in the elderly**, with great success. Tendinosis can be treated like any other tendinosis: exercises, light therapy, prolotherapy, PRP, etc. Diagnosis can be made via musculoskeletal ultrasound imaging or MRI. Along with the tendinosis/tendon tears, they may have other dysfunctional muscle activation patterns and the associated/corresponding muscle knots.

Lower cross syndrome

It is typical with pelvis/hip/knee issues for the glute med to be deactivated, but it isn't the only dysfunction. Often the TFL, lateral quads, psoas, and hamstrings are tight with glute max, glute med, medial quads, and the abs being deactivated. This results in the pelvis being tipped forward when standing: anterior pelvic tilt. I start with checking all the muscles for muscle knots, then I stretch the tight muscles. Then I exercise the deactivated muscles. It is debatable whether to start with a pure muscle building protocol (multiple sets at maximum difficulty with rest days to recover), or more rehab-type protocol (daily or multiple times a day sets that don't go all the way to muscle failure). Regardless of which strategy, people tend to improve. Reducing anterior tilt can prevent the muscle tension and muscle knots from returning. People often feel younger and taller and more fit (particularly if they can feel their ab muscles engaged).

Bad muscle activation patterns: Do you know how to use stairs?

You would be surprised how often people can't climb stairs properly. Whether from the fatigue of life as you age or from an injury, it can result in your hips sagging as you try to climb stairs. This results in a strain on the knee, the muscles along the outside of the thigh, and the hip musculature. Even when I demonstrate for patients what "wrong" looks like, it is very uncomfortable. I can feel the additional burden on the muscles and tendons, and it borders on pain. No wonder people who do it wrong have chronically painful hips and knees.

Correcting this can be a bit tricky. It takes babies months to learn how to walk and navigate stairs well. Relearning the coordination can be challenging, and sometimes there is muscle weakness to deal with as well (glute med!). Patients can get frustrated that they can't figure out how to get their hips to move how they want. This reprogramming can take days/weeks of practice to relearn how to do stairs properly.

First, I look at their hip levels as they go up a step. The hips should stay approximately level. If the hip drops and only gets lifted up right at the end, that is a bad sign. I will then break it down to the first part of the motion, just placing their foot onto a stair/step, ideally with a mirror so they can see their hips. Often their hip will already be in a dropped position. I have them square their hips. I then have them start to shift weight onto the leg on the step. Commonly, the hip will slip back to its habitual/wrong position. I have them reset and practice again, slowly, over sometimes multiple sessions, until they are able to step up without the hip dropping.

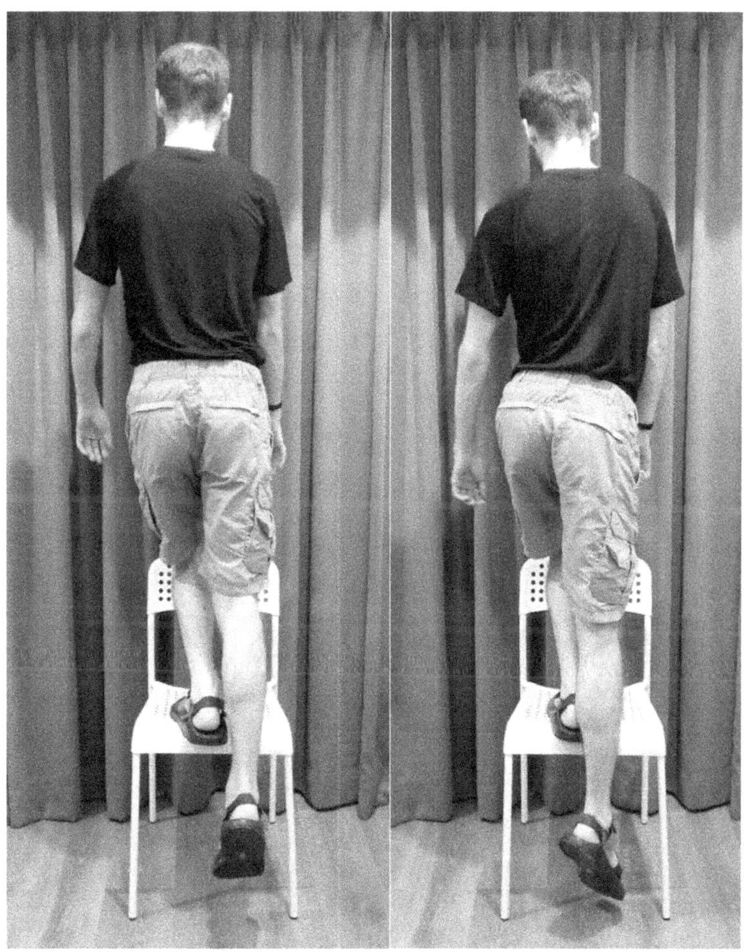

Can you walk properly?

Age or an injury (limping or crutch use) may affect your walk at the level of the hip or lower (read the ankle/foot section, too). When analyzing someone's gait, I start by looking at their hip: do they have equal sway to both sides, does the hip stick out to one side more than the other, are they leaning, is one leg/pelvis staying more flexed/bent than the other (asymmetric anterior pelvic tilt)?

The asymmetry could be from a muscle knot or scar tissue, so it is a good idea to check for muscle knots, scar tissue, and weak glute med even before checking gait. Next is either tightness and/or bad habits. Stretch anything too tight. Sometimes looong passive stretches. Gymnasts or dancers trying to achieve their splits don't hold their stretches for just a few seconds, they hold them for minutes. Having the patient stand and push their hips to either side, or hip thrust in the forward diagonals can reveal the tight spots. Sometimes patients struggle with getting their muscles to move their hips to one side. In that case, that is a strong indication of bad habits. Practicing "sassy" hips, hip thrusts, and/or walking with exaggerated hip sways can help with retraining. (It also never hurts to work on the core and glutes, too.)

KNEE

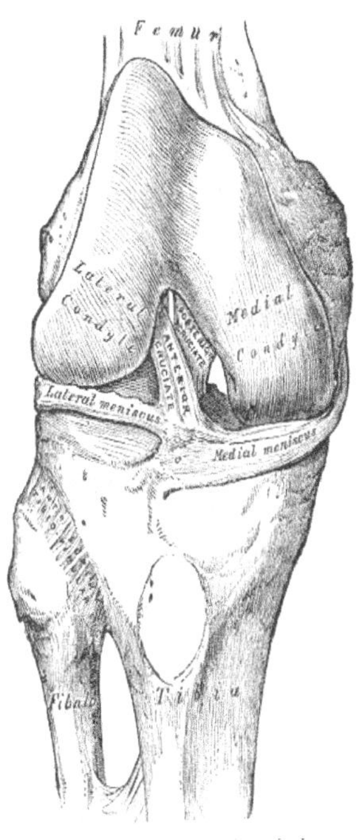

The knees take a lot of abuse and are the most common joints to be replaced (with hip being the second most common).[170] It is common for everyone to get osteoarthritis and weight, activity level, and previous injuries/surgeries influence the speed of degeneration. Like I've mentioned many times, arthritis ≠ pain (although it is possible to be causal/related). I recently had an active woman in her late 50s with chronic knee pain. With ultrasound imaging, I saw no cartilage left at all and thought, *If anybody's pain comes from arthritis, then it has got to be this woman's*. In defiance

[170] Singh JA. Epidemiology of knee and hip arthroplasty: a systematic review. *Open Orthop J.* 2011;5:80-85. Published 2011 Mar 16. doi:10.2174/1874325001105010080

of my hubris, that wasn't the case. I continued to image and I saw some funny looking (disorganized) tissue just behind the outside of her knee. It looked like scar tissue. Sure enough, pushing on it recreated her pain, and after I worked it out, she said her pain was completely gone and she could get back to her yoga pain-free. In pretty much every study on exercises (including squats) they found improvements in stiffness, pain, and function.[171,172] It doesn't have to be squats, as aquatic exercises, cycling, etc. can all be beneficial. Aren't exercises hard on the knee? If anything, the wear and tear on the knee should be worse, right? This goes to show that the pain isn't necessarily from the state of the knee (the arthritis). Also, having the muscles of your knee work well together can help minimize wear and tear forces on the knee.

Which tendons are prone to tendinosis?

The most common tendons prone to tendinosis is a set of tendons along the inside of the knee inserting just past the joint line called the pes anserinus (goose's foot) made up of the sartorius, gracilis, and semitendinosus tendons. The pes anserine bursa can also be a pain source and often this is diagnosed as a bursitis (acute bursal inflammation). In my clinical experience, when I do imaging, a tendinosis or tear

---

[171] Mo L, Jiang B, Mei T, Zhou D. Exercise Therapy for Knee Osteoarthritis: A Systematic Review and Network Meta-analysis. *Orthop J Sports Med.* 2023;11(5):23259671231172773. Published 2023 Jun 5. doi:10.1177/23259671231172773

[172] Raposo F, Ramos M, Lúcia Cruz A. Effects of exercise on knee osteoarthritis: A systematic review. *Musculoskeletal Care.* 2021;19(4):399-435. doi:10.1002/msc.1538

is more likely than a bursitis, but they are not mutually exclusive. It may be possible that even when the bursa has additional fluid, the pain is from a nearby tendon issue, like for the trochanteric bursa of the hip. The patellar tendon just below the kneecap is another possible tendinosis and/or gout location.

The tendinosis tendons will be tender to pressure and may be painful with use or extended use. Patellar tendinosis is more treated via exercise because it is easy to target. It gets used most as soon as you bend your knees while weight bearing. The pes anserinus is more challenging to treat via exercise, so I opt for all the other tendinosis treatments (red light, needling, PRP, etc.) combined with temporarily reducing aggravating activities.

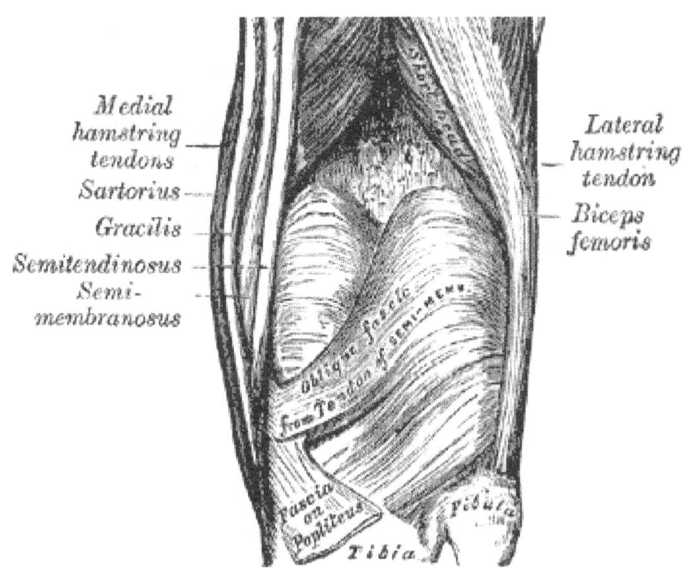

Is your knee pain coming from the hip/thigh?

Issues with the hips/pelvis can refer pain to the knee and/or can be the root cause of the knee problems. Muscle knots in the lateral glutes and/or TFL can refer to the posterior and lateral knee respectively. Nerve pain from a low back or a pelvic issue can also travel to any portion of the knee. Typically, referred pains are not precise in location, and a clue that your pain is referred is if you press where the pain is and it doesn't recreate/worsen it (although, if it is tender there you might have more than one issue). Bad walking (limping) and bad stair climbing habits (dropping the hip) can mess up the normal muscle functioning of the knee/hip and result in more wear and tear and more muscle knots. TFL muscle knots are often associated with vastus lateralis muscle knots and related to clicking knees. The vastus medialis and glute med might have to be reconditioned.

Clicking knees?

These are often non-painful but annoying. They may be associated with thigh/hip muscle knots and arthritis-type pain/pressure/swelling with lots of knee use, so sometimes the knee clicking can be related to knee pain. People might have clicking knees most of their life: with stairs, with squats, and with getting up. While grinding is more likely arthritis and locking may be loose pieces of bone or a torn meniscus, the typical clicking is from the patella (knee cap). It is a mismatch between the muscles that attach to the outside of the patella and the muscles that attach to the inside. You can imagine that if the muscles aren't pulling evenly, that that is going to mess up the biomechanics (how things work). Sometimes I feel the inside muscles (the vastus medialis) and they are half the size they should be! The outside muscles may be tight and full of muscle knots. The IT band and the vastus lateralis attach to the outside of the patella. The TFL is the main muscle that tenses the IT band. Read the hip section for more about TFL issues and the possible glute med weakness causing it. Vastus lateralis muscle knots tend to be in its upper two thirds. Special squats and knee extension exercises can target the inside knee muscles and can quickly recover the equilibrium between the inside and outside, often in a couple of weeks, in my experience. My go-to exercise is a squat which looks fairly normal, but as you do the squat, you try to twist your feet outwards unsuccessfully because of the friction between your feet and the floor (knees-over-toes is okay). You can even have your hands on your thighs, feeling for the increased muscle activation of the internal squad muscles.

Scar tissue and fascial adhesions

While I've already mentioned some knee pain might be muscles from the hip and in the ankle section, I will discuss muscle knots just below the knee joint that cause ankle pain. In addition to muscle knots, there is a similarly annoying and similarly treatable issue with the muscles that I find plagues legs/knees more than anywhere else on the body (except maybe the hands) and that is scar tissue and fascial adhesions. I wrote a section in the first part of the book, but I want to highlight it here specifically. Shake those individual hamstring muscles if they don't glide one on the other.

If it isn't a tear or fresh injury, then cross friction that painful spot. Push on the painful pinch location as you try to move. Breaking up the fascial adhesions and scar tissues can have immediate effects if this was the problem. I'm thinking of both a martial artist and a young sprinter who both complained that their legs were never being the same since they tore their hamstrings. After one session, they were basically back to normal again.

"But I tore my ACL, meniscus, etc."

Don't let old injuries keep you from trying to recondition the knee. While your knee might be a lost cause, I've seen plenty of knees recover without needing to resort to surgery. You have to give it a serious try. I'll give two examples.

I am the first example. I had a torn meniscus after being hit by a car. My knee wasn't painful, but there was a sense of pressure which worsened with activity, and the knee would lock. If your knee locks badly and continuously, consider a surgical consult. It basically kept me from cycling or doing stairs. I finally did the exercises seriously (despite them sometimes aggravating my knee) and was able to get back to all my activities without surgery, although I can still "feel" that knee a bit more than the other.

The second example is someone who complained of back and pelvis pain because he felt "twisted" ever since he tore his ACL more than 20 years previously and never had it surgically repaired. I went and checked his knees. The right one had a little bit of extra motion, but was still within normal, and the left one was rock-solid, indicating a tight/strong ACL. Well, it turns out it was the left one he had torn and, not only did it fix itself, but it was now even tighter than his right ACL! In fact, ACLs can spontaneously heal, and it is debated whether you should repair it right away or wait to see if it fixes itself.[173] Anyways, I looked at his quads and the left was significantly smaller. He had basically stopped all activities that would have stressed his knee since the injury more than 20 years ago. Starting to use that knee again would be the long-term solution to his pelvic/hip issues.

When should I get knee surgery or a knee replacement?

When should you go for knee replacements, ACL repairs, meniscectomies, etc.? The strongest indicators are if the joint is swollen, locking, giving way, and/or losing range of motion. Be sure to investigate all the other sources of pain as you can have more than one type/source of pain.

---

[173] Blanke F, Trinnes K, Oehler N, et al. Spontaneous healing of acute ACL ruptures: rate, prognostic factors and short-term outcome. *Arch Orthop Trauma Surg.* 2023;143(7):4291-4298. doi:10.1007/s00402-022-04701-0

ANKLE/FOOT

Ankle/Foot pain is a tricky one, in part because if problems have persisted long enough, sometimes there is no reversing the issue. That being said, it isn't all doom and gloom. There are plenty of cases of chronic ankle clicking/discomfort or people's chronic "plantar fasciitis" that I've resolved in a visit or two! In addition to physical therapists and chiropractors, with feet, you have access to professionals who specialize in just foot problems: podiatrists/chiropodists.

Muscle knots!

Always with the muscle knots! Most ankle and foot/toe muscles are quite long and are located in the calf. In particular, it tends to be the upper calf (outside/lateral more than inside/medial), sometimes surprisingly close to the knee. Like in other instances, you are looking for traveling pain towards the ankle/foot and/or a recreation of your pain with compression. For the calf, like the forearm, I find dry needling a little more effective than ischemic compression, but both work for the upper half of the calf. I find compression works best at the bottom of the foot. The muscle knots at the bottom of the foot can mimic a chronic "plantar fasciitis."

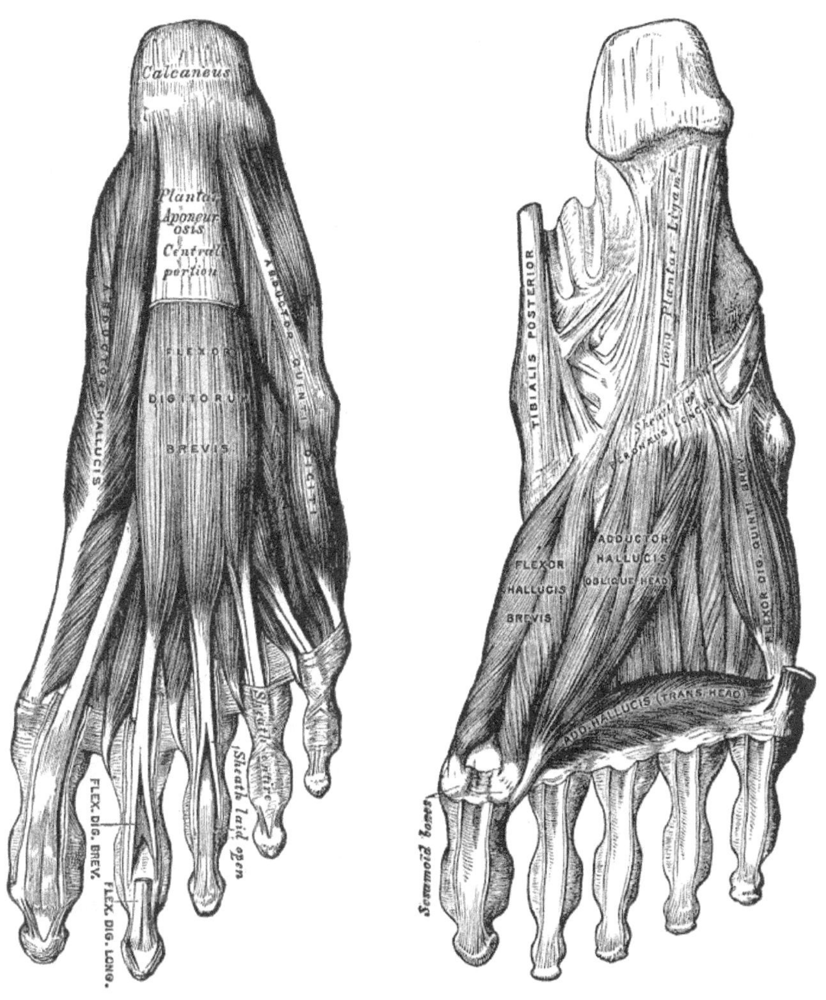

Acquired flat feet? Pain on the inside of the arch?

If you haven't always had flat feet but acquired them later in life, then chances are you have fully torn a tendon on the inside of your foot that helps hold the arch up. If you still have your arch but currently have pain on the inside of your arch, then it could be that same tendon is tearing and/or weakening.

One of the most common tendon issues in the ankle/foot are issues with the posterior tibial tendon (that holds up the arch of the foot).[174] The attached muscle is called the tibialis posterior. Problems with this tendon are sometimes called posterior tibial tendon dysfunction. Problems with this tendon are often misdiagnosed. In fact, it is hard to get a number for how often it may be misdiagnosed or what percentage of people will get it (incidence rate) since it is misdiagnosed so often. In one study, they found that 88% of patients were initially misdiagnosed, and waited an average of 43 months to receive the correct diagnosis.[175] Risk factors include being over the age of fifty, obesity, ankle trauma, and local steroid injections. This tendon runs behind the medial malleolus (the bony part that juts out on the inside of the ankle). It then runs under the arch. The rupture can happen suddenly but normally a tendinosis leads up to the rupture. The tendon pain of the tendinosis can mimic an ankle sprain, Achilles tendon pain, or plantar fasciitis pain.

If the tendinosis progresses, then the tendon may fully rupture. Once this occurs, your arch will flatten out, and you will have acquired a flat foot. There is good news, though, that the surgery to repair this tendon has a high success rate.

---

[174] Knapp PW, Constant D. Posterior Tibial Tendon Dysfunction. [Updated 2023 May 23]. In: StatPearls [Internet]. Treasure Island (FL): *StatPearls Publishing*; 2023 Jan. Available from: https://www.ncbi.nlm.nih.gov/books/NBK542160/

[175] Mann FA, Thompson FM. Rupture of the posterior tibial tendon causing flatfoot. *J Bone Joint Surg* 1985;67A:556–61.

Confirmatory diagnosis of posterior tibial tendon dysfunction can very accurately and quickly be done through musculoskeletal ultrasound.[176] If the tendinosis is treated via PRP, prolotherapy, light therapy, exercises, etc., you may avoid a full rupture and the need for surgery.

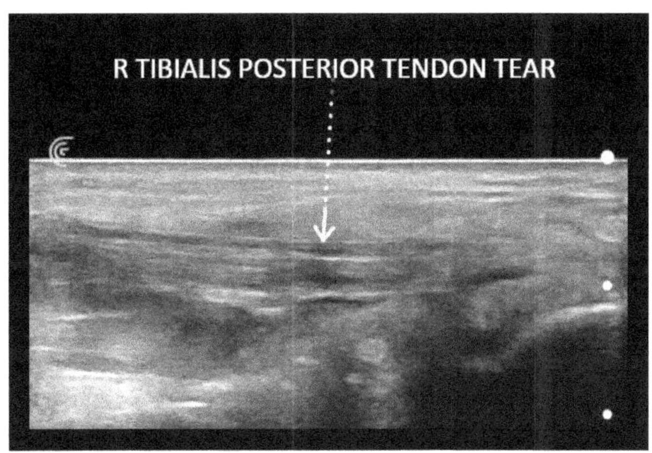

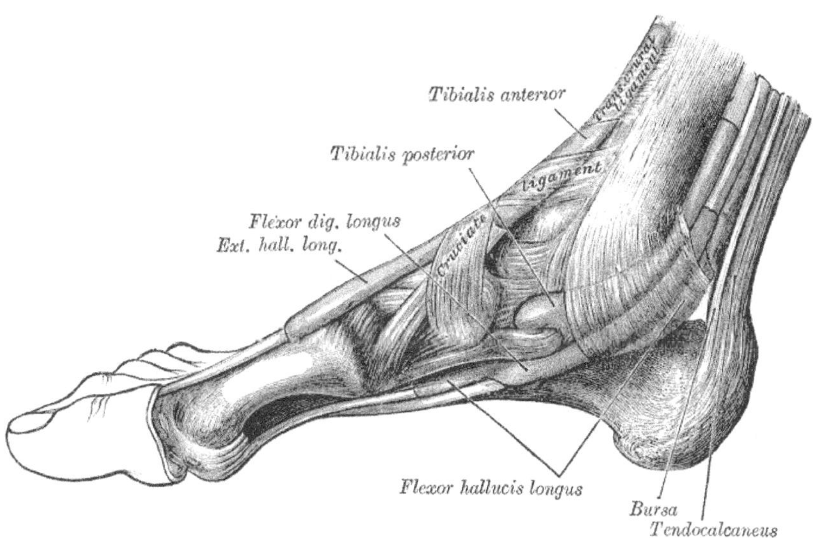

---

[176] Ramakko B, Point-of-Care Musculoskeletal Ultrasound in the Diagnosis of Tibialis Posterior Partial Tendon Tear: A Case Report. *J Int Acad Neuromusculoskel Med.* 2022 Dec;19(2):2-6

Achilles tendon pain?

The Achilles tendon (labeled tendocalcaneus in the nearby images) connects the largest muscles of the calf to the heel. Chronic pain here is less common than at the plantar fascia or the posterior tibial tendon. It could be muscle knots in the calf, scar tissue, fascial adhesions, or muscle herniations. An ultrasound can quickly and easily evaluate for tendinosis and most other pathologies. The scar tissue/adhesions can be worked out with X-friction massage and/or by vigorously moving the tissue. Ischemic compression or dry needling can be done for the muscle knots, and eccentric exercises/red light therapy/PRP/etc. can be done for a tendinosis.

The Achilles tendon is readily treated through exercises. Our muscles are stronger as they lengthen instead of when shortening, and we want the force into our tendon, not necessarily our muscles, which is why eccentric (as the muscle is lengthening) is normally the exercise of choice as it is easiest on ourselves and our muscles. In some studies, the exact type of exercise (eccentric, concentric, isometric) might not matter as much.[177]

Now to describe the exercise and to tailor it to your ability. Pain for tendinosis shouldn't be more than a 3/10. Choose a step. Place yourself such that your heels are just off the back of the step. Raise up with both feet on your tip toes but come

[177] Gatz M, Betsch M, Dirrichs T, et al. Eccentric and Isometric Exercises in Achilles Tendinopathy Evaluated by the VISA-A Score and Shear Wave Elastography. *Sports Health.* 2020;12(4):373-381. doi:10.1177/1941738119893996

back down slowly with most (or all) your weight on the symptomatic side. Repeat 3 sets of 10. The reason a step is used is that it allows for a greater range of motion. You can make the exercise easier by not using a step, by using both feet for up and down, by reducing reps/sets, and/or by holding onto a counter/doing it seated. To increase the challenge you can add weights, add a quick rebound at the bottom, and/or by using just one leg for both up and down.[178]

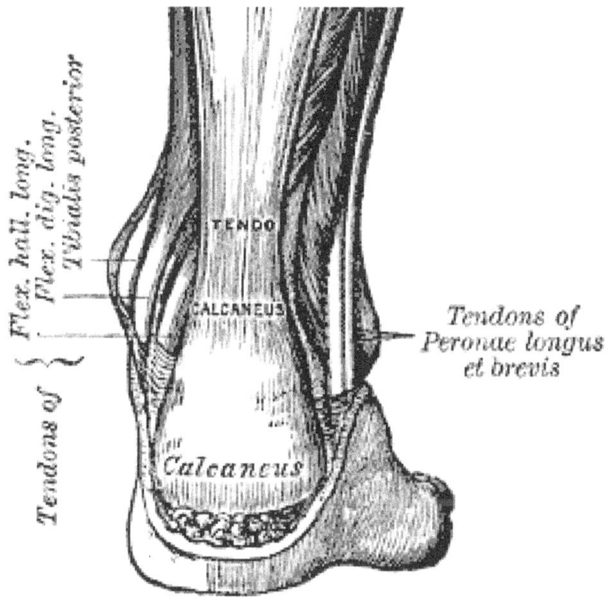

Chronic "plantar fasciitis"?

The plantar fascia acts as a broad tendon/ligament along the bottom of the foot. It is prone to the same issues as any tendon, and so "chronic plantar fasciitis" is the equivalent condition to a tendinosis (degenerative rather than acute),

---

[178] "Achilles Tendinopathy Toolkit: Section D - Exercise Programs." *Physiopedia*, . 3 Dec 2022, https://www.physio-pedia.com/Achilles_Tendinopathy_Toolkit:_Section_D_-_Exercise_Programs

and it should more accurately called a plantar fasciosis. This correct term is so rarely used that I even find myself using plantar fasciitis when I'm rushed and I don't have to explain myself. It is very easily diagnosed accurately via ultrasound. Interestingly, since I have started using musculoskeletal ultrasound in practice, I diagnose this much less than I thought as most pain has been muscle knots at the bottom of the foot! Even if it isn't the muscles at the bottom of the foot, the foot pain could be from a posterior tibial tendinosis, scar tissue, bones out of alignment, nerve pain, muscle knots in the calf, etc. The nerves could be also be pinched at the ankle or the knee, but that pain tends to be more burning, tingling, and numb.

Plantar fasciosis can be treated like any other tendinosis. The symptoms tend to be pain mostly upon standing first thing in the morning. The windlass test is fairly helpful. You push on the front inside of the heel, then with your other hand, bend the big toe up. If moving the big toe increases pain then that suggests plantar fasciosis. In addition to the typical tendinosis treatments, "tear-drop" style athletic taping can help relieve symptoms and wearing a boot/brace that keeps the foot neutral instead of pointed during sleep can help. The idea behind the brace being that, since fasciosis is microtears the body is trying to heal, if it heals overnight with the foot pointed, the fascia healed shortened. First thing in the morning when you try to stretch it, you end up tearing the newly made repairs which causes the intense pain for the first few steps in the morning.

Nerve pain in the calf/foot?

As briefly mentioned when talking about plantar fasciosis, nerve compression/irritation can cause burning, shooting/electrical pain, numbness, tingling, and even weakness. The location of the nerve pinching is often not obvious and may be in multiple locations similar as was discussed for hand nerve symptoms. Hand nerve symptoms could be from an issue in the wrist, forearm, clavicle region, or neck and foot symptoms could be from a nerve issue at the foot, ankle, knee, pelvis, or spine. As mentioned elsewhere in this book, nerve symptoms may be from a systemic issue like a vitamin B12 deficiency or diabetes. Diabetes in particular starts to affect the feet first, then the hands and front/lateral thigh second. Diabetes leg/foot symptoms can lead to amputation!

Assuming the nerve symptoms are coming from nerve irritation/compression, then the issue could be at the spinal canal involving the discs or joints, an irritated sacroiliac (pelvis) joint, the piriformis muscle (in your butt/gluteal region), just past the knee joint (proximal tibia-fibula joint), or at the ankle. You could have issues with one region or multiple regions making the situation even more complicated. For the issues involving the spine and the pelvis, read the back and hip sections. We'll focus here on the nerve issues that occur past the knee.

The sciatic nerve that exits the pelvis splits into smaller nerves at the knee. One of these smaller nerves goes around the outside of the leg close to the proximal tibia-fibula joint. Sometimes crossing your legs can put pressure on the nerve and can squeeze it against the bone there. With extended cross-legged sessions, anyone might get tingles and numbness traveling down the calf to the outside and/or top of the foot. If it is very sensitive there, then maybe there are issues there. I've had some success in this region with mobilizing this joint with a quick thrust or gently shifting it back and forth. Working out any muscle knots in the proximity, cupping, and/or needling has also helped. A reminder that not all strategies work on every patient as everyone's problems are unique.

At the ankle there is a region analogous to the carpal tunnel for the wrist called the tarsal tunnel. Both structures are tunnels through which arteries, veins, tendons, and nerves travel. Both are contained by a retinaculum, a ligament-like structure that acts as the roof of the tunnel holding everything in. If there is something taking up space in the tunnel, like a swollen tendon, it can limit the space within the tunnel. The nerve could be more prone to irritation in this region due to activities, weight, choice of footwear, loss of arch, and habits. Regardless of the reason, the nerve can be evaluated directly using ultrasound imaging. The pain/burning/tingling/numbness pattern is often the inside and bottom of the foot. If someone taps over the tarsal tunnel and it causes shooting pain (Tinel's test/sign) on the bottom of your foot, that is also suggestive that you have nerve pain. If it exactly reproduces your complaint, then you don't have "chronic plantar fasciitis."

Ankle "pinching" or clicking?

This can be from a few issues. This could be from tight/painful scar tissue. Working out the scar tissue might be the solution. Otherwise, this may require tweaks to the joint to get things working well again: a chiropractor might say, "to re-align things." This might be joint mobilizations, stretches, and exercises. I worked with a 36-year-old with two clicky ankles since childhood. They would click with almost every step. I did a quick pull on both of them and they've been silent ever since.

Sharp pinching pain in the foot?

Foot pinching may be similar to ankle pinching. There are tiny bones between the main ankle joint and the main long bones of the foot. These can be painfully "misaligned." Sometimes exercises and mobilizing helps. Sometimes the displacement is too severe and surgery may be a reasonable option.

There is a nerve issue that can result in sharp burning nerve pain between the toes called a Morton's neuroma. This is a painful and swollen nerve that appears as a small ball of nerve tissue on ultrasound imaging. Normally these are found between the bony metatarsal heads at the bases of the toes, in one of the center two spaces. You can imagine that with each step, the nerve may be aggravated, and the pain may be intense. If it isn't too bad then rest, losing weight, and avoiding aggravating factors (like high heels) might be sufficient. If the pain is severe and/or the problem is not resolving then steroid/cortisone injections, radio-ablation (nerve destruction), or surgery can be considered. A test for this is called the metatarsal squeeze test, or Morton's test, where you squeeze all the bases of the toes from the sides. If this increases pain, that may be a positive, but even more so if you hear a click, which is called Mulder's sign. The click is from the swollen nerve being squished out from between the bone spaces.

Ankle locking?

Floating bone pieces may be the culprit. X-rays or CT scans may find them. This may be from late-stage osteoarthritis and may indicate time for an ankle replacement or at least surgical removal of the bone fragments. A blocked sensation at the extremes of motion can be from osteoarthritis (bone spurs) but it also might be something simple like a tightness or misalignment which may be resolved by mobilizing the ankle joint, the smaller bones of the foot, and/or stretching the calf.

Chronic ankle sprains and ankle instability?

Spraining your ankle once more than doubles your chances of spraining it again.[179] A whopping 40% of people who sprain their ankle go on to have chronic issues that persist more than 12 months: swelling, pain, instability, and more ankle sprains![180]

---

[179] Delahunt E, Remus A. Risk Factors for Lateral Ankle Sprains and Chronic Ankle Instability. *J Athl Train.* 2019;54(6):611-616. doi:10.4085/1062-6050-44-18

[180] Chen ET, Borg-Stein J, McInnis KC. Ankle Sprains: Evaluation, Rehabilitation, and Prevention [published correction appears in Curr Sports Med Rep. 2019 Aug;18(8):310]. *Curr Sports Med Rep.* 2019;18(6):217-223. doi:10.1249/JSR.0000000000000603

With any sprain, you may have muscle spasms protecting the joint. From the limping and protecting you may develop bad muscle habits. Combine both of these, and you have a recipe for muscle knots in the calf. Repaired tissue can be disorganized and more painful. Breaking up scar tissue if present can be key to reducing sharp pain persisting past the initial recovery period.

Let's talk about ankle stability. After a leg injury, you may use the foot less and maybe you alter how you walk for a while. This results in a loss of muscle control and proprioception (your body's ability to know where the joint is). The less-used muscles may also have become weak. Typical rehab is using a TheraBand (exercise band) to work out the muscles in 3 of the 4 directions (up, inwards/pronation, outwards/eversion) and for the 4th direction to use calf raises (going onto your toes). This all works for the strength aspect. But what about proprioception and control? Typically, the patient works through variations of standing on one leg: eyes open vs closed, flat ground vs unsteady surface, still vs hopping, and without moving vs slowly moving arms or legs to shift weight. Once you feel your balance is reasonable, the rehab is over.

Do you walk funny?

Through lack of activity for years or after an injury (limping or crutch use) your walking gait may have developed some bad habits at the level of the hip (read the hip section) or lower. After checking the hips while analyzing gait, I set my sights lower. I focus on their knees, ankles, and feet. Do they hyperextend one or both knees? Is one leg more externally rotated than the other. Do the feet have equal symmetry? Do they toe-off (push off) properly? Most commonly I see a lack of proper toe-off. You should strike with the outside heel, then the weight shifts toward the mid toes before ending up at the base of the big toe for pushing off. This is trickier to fix than the hip issues as there is a lot more variety in "correct" and there is also the fact that "how good can it get" could be limited considering the history of leg/foot injuries.

What are "Good Shoes"?

This could be a book in itself. For different people, with different genetics, and different issues, and for different purposes, the definition of a good shoe will vary. Let's talk about bad shoes first, because that is easier. High heels are awful. Although some level of heel lift in shoes can be beneficial in some cases, I recommend little to no heel lift (0-10mm). The toe box should mimic your natural toe shape as much as possible, but the common shape in the shoe industry is too pointy: the big toes and little toes are pushed inward unnaturally, resulting in deformities over time. If your feet are now misshapen, then maybe that shape of running/walking shoe is comfortable but, in general, a shoe where the peak is between the big toe and first normal toe (labeled digits 1 and 2 in anatomy) is best for the feet. Try on lots of shoes and pick the ones that fit and feel the best to move around in. Wearing good socks too is good advice in general (try merino wool).

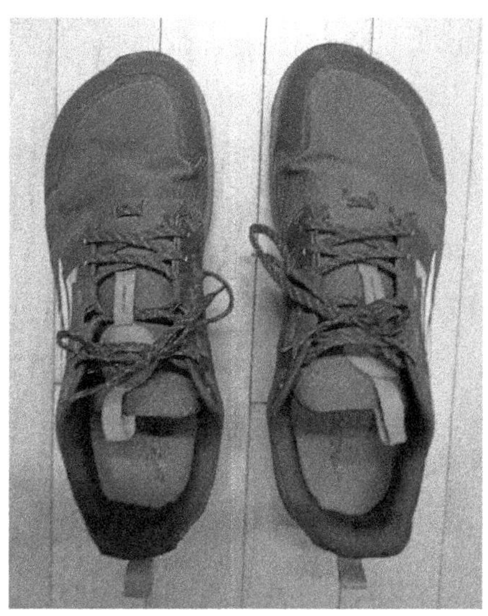

Do you need custom orthotics? Should the arch support be significant?

I touched on this briefly in the chapter on braces. Our feet weren't designed for shoes. The muscles and joints are designed for the weight to rest on the ball of the foot and the heel. A custom arch, or a high arch, that takes up the arch space changes how your foot works. While it may help, it can irritate the joints, anger some muscles, and weaken others. If you've ruptured the tibialis posterior tendon and lost your arch (consider surgery!) then forcing an arch might be better than the alternative. Custom orthotics or off the shelf inserts are something I consider with patients for foot, knee, and/or hip issues that are fairly persistent but they are things to experiment with, not something set in stone. I've seen it make patients worse! There can be a perverse incentive in healthcare when there is profit to be made. I regularly get emails and flyers touting how much more money I'd bring in by selling custom orthotics but I am currently not interested as I get fairly good results without selling them.

Do you have big toe pain?

That poor big toe. It is arguably the most prone to osteoarthritis pain and years of bad shoe use can leave the joints dysfunctional and painful. Autoimmune arthritis loves to attack it too, but I won't delve into the autoimmune stuff in this book. I will, however, cover a couple structural issues, their possible solutions, and I'll briefly cover gout again.

The big toe is typically the first place that gout appears. Gout is when uric acid crystals start to form in joints and tendons. These crystals are like sharp ninja stars or caltrops. The joint becomes red, hot, burning, stiff, and very sensitive to touch. The elbow or knee joints are some of the next most common locations. It is from an overconsumption of purine rich foods. Chronic/recurrent gout can be a diet issue or an organ issue with how your body is eliminating the uric acid from the body. There are drugs that can help with the body's processing, but diet is the first line treatment for eliminating acute and/or returning gout by reducing the consumption of purine rich foods (seafood, alcohol, etc.) and overly sweetened products (fructose ultimately gets broken down into uric acid).

A stiff, bony, big toe is called "hallux rigidus." This is our friend osteoarthritis and it can be painful with use. While I have explained that arthritis can be considered normal, age-related bony changes, the wear and tear at the toe joint can be greatly accelerated by genetic predisposition, history of injuries, and bad footwear. If the biomechanics can still be changed, maybe through better shoes, then there is a chance of reversal of the pain and symptoms of hallux rigidus. There are surgical options once the toe is unusable and/or the pain becomes too much.

Related to hallux rigidus are bunions. Bunions (a bump on the inside-base of the big toe) are often found combined with hallux valgus (hallux means big toe and valgus means displaced from the midline of the body), where the big toe is pushed towards the center of the foot. Some people are more genetically predisposed to developing this deformity as they use their feet over the decades but...

RANT INCOMING: Call me a conspiracy theorist if you must, but I think there is a movement to shift the blame away from footwear. If you google "bunions," "high heels," or "narrow shoes" there will be lots of articles on how high heels don't cause bunions, the shoes just exacerbate the problem. The real cause is the person, not the shoes. The person must have a genetic predisposition. They must have previous injuries. I believe this is mostly bullshit. Men rarely get bunions. Women who wear comfy shoes their whole life rarely get them either, but women who wear high heels always seem to have bunions in my clinical experience. This scenario reminds me of type-2 diabetes where, at least in the states, they blame genetic factors, but not diet. Research will show that even for those with genetic predispositions, individuals on plant-based diets won't get type-2 diabetes, and early type-2 diabetes is reversible through diet alone. People just want to still wear their high heels and narrow shoes and companies are happy to still keep selling them. People

still want to overeat and eat sweet things. Society is in de-
nial!

RANT OVER. Long story short, if you have bunions wear
more comfortable shoes. If you are a woman and worried
you might get bunions, start wearing the comfiest, least
pointy shoes you can get. Treatment for bunions and hallux
valgus include joint manipulation and exercises by a
physio/chiro/podiatrist, orthotics, bunion pads, taping, toe
spacers, good shoes, and, ultimately, surgery.

ABOUT THE AUTHOR

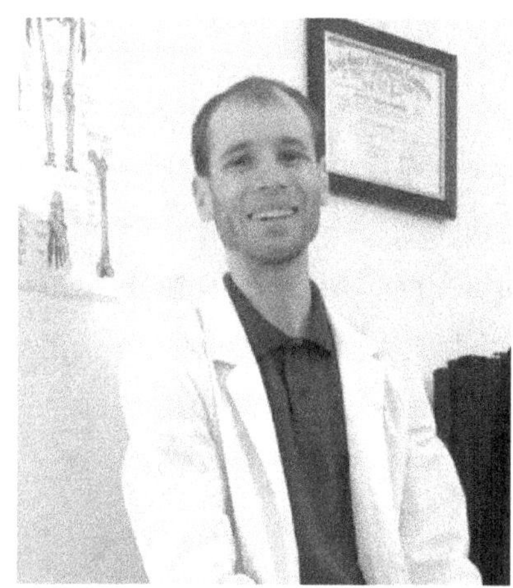

Dr. Ramakko spent most of his adult life teaching college-level physics in Montreal, Canada, but when his own health and the health of his loved ones declined due to indifferent and unsatisfactory healthcare, he took it upon himself to start his own healthcare education. He tries to share this knowledge as much as possible. He is unsatisfied with people's health being "good enough" and strives to get patients feeling their best and optimizing their quality of life. While happy to work with a variety of conditions, he has particular interest in chronic pain. To find out more or to book a session with him you can go to www.DrRamakko.com

Some highlights:

DIANM: Diplomate Status with the International Academy of Neuromusculoskeletal medicine indicating expertise in diagnosis and management as a "neuromusculoskeletal medicine specialist."

RMSK: "Registered in Musculoskeletal Sonography" indicating expertise in taking and interpreting diagnostic musculoskeletal ultrasound images.

DipIBLM: Board certified "Lifestyle Medicine professional." Advises patients in lifestyle interventions to treat, prevent, and/or reverse relevant chronic diseases.

As an Educator: Previously a full-time college physics teacher for seven years including serving as curriculum coordinator. Also holds a "Higher Education Teaching Certificate" from Harvard and a TEFL certificate.

As a Chiropractor: Trained in Oregon at University of Western States (UWS) as a primary care practitioner. Graduated "summa cum laude." Worked in his own practice in Texas and at a multidisciplinary clinic in the Cayman Islands. Trained in Acupuncture (Passed the NBCE acupuncture exam).

As a Researcher: Published seven peer-reviewed articles (mostly in physics).